W0043299

To Hilde, Sarah and Ine

W. Flameng (Ed.)

Temporary Cardiac Assist with an Axial Pump System

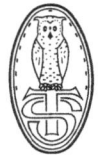 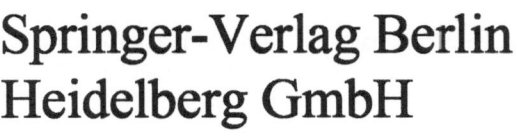 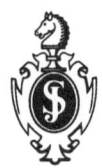

Springer-Verlag Berlin
Heidelberg GmbH

Editor:

Willem Flameng M.D.
Department of Cardiac Surgery
Katholieke Universiteit Leuven
B-3000 Leuven
Belgium

Cover illustration:
Study of Archimedes's screw-driven
water pump by Leonardo da Vinci,
ca. 1475–80.
Milan, Ambrosiana, Codex Atlanticus

Die Deutsche Bibliothek – CIP-Einheitsaufnahme

Temporary cardiac assist with an axial pump system / W.
Flameng (ed.).

   ISBN 978-3-7985-0906-1   ISBN 978-3-662-10284-8 (eBook)
   DOI 10.1007/978-3-662-10284-8
NE: Flameng, Willem [Hrsg.]

This work is subject to copyright. All rights are reserved whether the whole or part of the material is concerned, specifically the rights of translation, reprinting, re-use of illustrations, recitations, broadcasting, reproduction on microfilms or in other ways, and storage in data banks. Duplication of this publication or parts thereof is only permitted under the provision of the German Copyright Law of September 9, 1965, in its version of June 24, 1985, and a copyright fee must always be paid. Violations fall under the prosecution act of the German Copyright Law.

Copyright © 1991 by Springer-Verlag Berlin Heidelberg
        Originally published by Dr. Dietrich Steinkopff Verlag GmbH & Co. KG, Darmstadt in 1991

Medical Editorial: Sabine Müller – English Editor: James C. Willis – Production: Heinz J. Schäfer

The use of registered names, trademarks, etc., in this publication does not imply, even in the absence of a specific statement, that such names are exempt from the relevant protective laws and regulations and therefore free for general use.

Type-setting,
Printed on acid-free paper

Preface

With this book, it was not our intention to provide a complete "textbook" on axial pumps and their use as temporary cardiac assist systems. It is more a sharing of experiences with a novel left-ventricular assist system, the Hemopump, as it was developed by R. K. Wampler. This device, marketed by Johnson & Johnson Interventional Systems, has not yet been widely used and accepted in clinical practice. It was offered to us some time ago to study its applicability in the experimental setting. At the moment, it is under investigation in many centers and it is commercially available. However, as with any other cardiac assist system, the axial pump has its own advantages and limitations. Needless to say, critical analysis of such a novel device is mandatory and, therefore, we are grateful to our colleagues who were willing to contribute to this book. They present, discuss, and analyze their experimental and clinical experience with the Hemopump and focus on side-effects, deficiency and efficiency of this device which, by virtue of its simplicity is revolutionary.

Leuven, Belgium, 1991   Willem Flameng

Contributors

H. Reul, Ph.D.
Helmholtz Institute for Biomedical Engineering at the RWTH Aachen, Pauwelstrasse 30,
D-5100 Aachen, FRG

R.K. Wampler, M.D.
Nimbus Medical, Inc., 2890 Kilgore Road, Rancho Cordova, California 95670, USA

K.-H. Scholz, M.D.
Kliniken der Universität Göttingen, Fachbereich Medizin, Zentrum Innere Medizin
Abt. Kardiologie, Robert Kochstrasse 40, D-3400 Göttingen, FRG

P. Wouters, M.D.
University Clinic Gasthuisberg, Department of Anesthesiology, Herestraat 49,
B-3000 Leuven, Belgium

O.H. Frazier, M.D.
Texas Heart Institute, 1101 Bates Avenue, Suite P-306, Houston, Texas 77030, USA

U. Mees, M.D.
University Clinic Gasthuisberg, Department of Cardiac Surgery, Herestraat 49,
B-3000 Leuven, Belgium

O. Jegaden, M.D.
Hôpital Vasculaire Louis Pradel, 59 Boulevard Pinel, F-69003 Lyon, France

D. Loisance, Ph.D., M.D.
Centre Hospitalier Henri Mondor, Faculté de Médecine, 8 Rue du Général Sarail,
F-94010 Créteil Cedex, France

W. Flameng, Ph.D., M.D.
University Clinic Gasthuisberg, Department of Cardiac Surgery, Herestraat 49,
B-3000 Leuven, Belgium

Contents

I. Basic Aspects

Hydromechanical principles of axial pumps

H. Reul

Helmholtz Institute for Biomedical Engineering, Aachen, FRG

Introduction

Generally, pumps can be classified into two main categories: displacement pumps and rotary pumps. The energy transfer in displacement pumps is characterized by periodic changes of a working space. Typical displacement pump types are piston pumps, gear pumps or roller pumps.

In rotary pumps the energy transfer to the fluid is due to velocity deflections within the impeller vanes. It can also be generally stated that for large volume flows and low pressures the advantages of rotary pumps predominate, while for low volume flows and high pressures displacement pumps are more suitable in most cases.

In the medical arena displacement type pumps (roller pumps) have been well established over decades in heart lung or dialysis machines. Their main advantages are simplicity of operation, low cost of disposable tubing, and reliability, whereas disadvantages can be seen in blood damage and spallation of tubing.

Due to several theoretical and practical advantages of rotary pumps in terms of lower blood damage, smaller size, lower filling volume, better transportability, and absence of spallation, a number of rotary pump types has been introduced for medical applications in recent years. All of them were of the centrifugal type and intended for extracorporeal use.

The first axial type blood pump is a very recent development and was introduced by Dr. Richard Wampler as an intraarterial miniature circulatory support system.

To give a better understanding of the working principle of rotary pumps, especially axial pumps, the following simplified engineering considerations may be of some value for the interested reader.

How does a rotary pump generate pressure?

Let us start with the well known Newton's law which describes the correlation between mass (m), velocity (v), and force (F):

$$F = \frac{d(m\,v)}{dt} \tag{1}$$

In solid body mechanics, where the mass of the body does not change, this law is usually written in the form:

$$F = m\frac{\delta v}{\delta t} = mass \cdot acceleration \tag{1a}$$

3

In case of a continuously working pump, however, where we have a mass flow, the local acceleration is zero, i.e., at a specific location the velocity does not change with time.

Then we may write Newton's law in the form:

$$F = m\frac{\delta m}{\delta t} \cdot v = m \cdot v = I = \text{momentum flux} = \text{force} \tag{2}$$

If this momentum flux is multiplied by a distance (d):

$$\dot{I} \cdot d = \dot{D} \tag{3}$$

it is called the moment of momentum, which is equal to a torque.

The resulting torque (M) which is exerted on a fluid by a rotating impeller can thus be written as the difference between $\dot{D}$ at the impeller exit minus $\dot{D}$ at the impeller inlet.

$$M = \dot{D}_{ex} - \dot{D}_{in}. \tag{4}$$

The torque is calculated with the circumferential components (c_u) of the absolute fluid velocities. The meridian components (c_m) do not contribute (see Fig. 1).

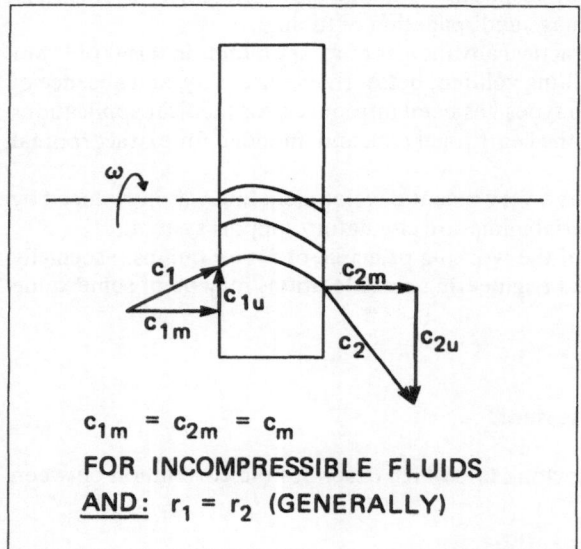

Fig. 1. Components of absolute velocity c for axial pumps.

For axial pumps the inlet radius (r_1) is equal to the exit radius (r_2) and the meridian components (c_m) are constant for incompressible fluids.

With (4), we then can write:

$$M = \dot{m} \cdot r\,(c_{2u} \cdot c_{1u}); \tag{5}$$

the transferred power is equal to the torque multiplied by the angular velocity (ω).

4

$$N = M \cdot \omega \tag{6}$$

and with (5):

$$N = \dot{m} \cdot \omega \cdot r \, (c_{2u} \cdot c_{1u}) \tag{7}$$

Since $\omega \cdot r$ is the circumferential velocity u, it follows that:

$$N = \dot{m} \cdot u \, (c_{2u} \cdot c_{1u}) \tag{8}$$

Correlation of power and generated pressure

Pressure is defined as energy per volume unit:

$$\text{pressure} \triangleq \frac{\text{energy}}{\text{volume unit}}$$

Based on this definition we can also write:

$$\text{pressure} \triangleq \frac{\text{energy/time unit}}{\text{volume unit/time unit}} \triangleq \frac{\text{power}}{\text{volume flow}} \, .$$

We thus can write:

$$\Delta p = \frac{N}{\dot{V}} \tag{9}$$

or:

$$N = \dot{V} \cdot \Delta p. \tag{10}$$

Combining (8) and (10), it follows that:

$$\dot{V} \cdot \Delta p = \dot{m} \cdot u \, (c_{2u} \cdot c_{1u}),$$

and with $\dot{m} = \dot{V} \cdot \rho$, we obtain the well-known Euler-equation for axial pumps:

$$\Delta p = \rho \cdot u \, (c_{2u} \cdot c_{1u}), \tag{11}$$

or, with $\Delta p = \rho \cdot g \cdot H$ in different form:

$$H = \frac{u}{g} \, (c_{2u} \cdot c_{1u}), \tag{12}$$

where H is the generated pressure head.

5

If we relate the transferred power $\dot{V} \cdot \Delta p$ to the mass flow $\dot{m}$, we obtain the so-called specific flow work y:

$$\frac{\dot{V} \cdot \Delta p}{\dot{m}} = u\,(c_{2u} - c_{1u}) = \frac{\Delta p}{\rho} = g \cdot H = y. \tag{13}$$

Some important characteristic dimensionless quantities:

– Related to pump characteristics

1) Head coefficient ψ: ψ relates the generated pressure head H to the dynamic impeller pressure.

$$\psi = \frac{\Delta p}{\frac{\rho}{2}\,u^2} = \frac{2gH}{u^2} = \frac{2y}{u^2} \tag{14}$$

2) Capacity coefficient ϕ: ϕ relates the meridian component of the absolute velocity to the circumferential velocity of the impeller.

$$\phi = \frac{c_m}{u} \tag{15}$$

– Related to pump type

1) Specific diameter δ: δ relates the outer diameter D of the impeller to the diameter of

a fictive nozzle with the same flow V and the same pressure head H.

$$\delta = 1.054 \cdot D \cdot \frac{y^{1/4}}{\dot{V}^{1/2}} \tag{16}$$

2) Specific speed σ: σ relates the rotational speed n to the rotational speed of a geometrically similar pump which delivers a unit flow at a unit pressure and a unit gravity.

$$\sigma = 2.108 \cdot n \cdot \frac{\dot{V}^{1/2}}{y^{3/4}} \tag{17}$$

Cordier diagram

The Cordier diagram (Fig. 2) shows the correlation of the above-listed dimensionless parameters. It was developed by O. Cordier, who correlated the calculated specific diameters δ of turbomachines with experimentally determined high efficiencies as a function of the specific speed σ. Each range of the diagram can be correlated to a typical pump – or turbine type. For example, all high-efficiency axial pumps lie in range 3 of this diagram.

6

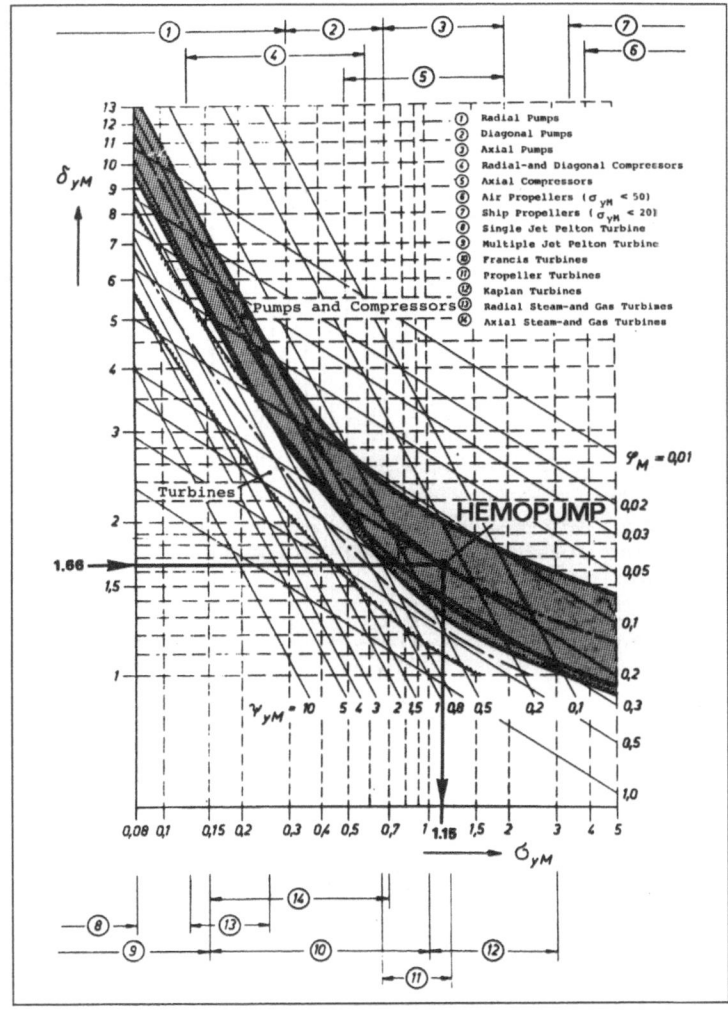

Fig. 2. Cordier diagram for turbomachines.

The Cordier diagram is the most valuable tool for the design of turbo-machines.

Fig. 3 shows the efficiency distribution over specific speed for turbo-machines, where curve 2 represents axial pumps.

Fig. 4 gives an overview of different impeller shapes from the radial to the axial pumps and the correlated specific speed and specific diameter.

Practical design considerations

Let us now apply the above basic engineering principles to the design of the Hemopump, as an example.

We want to develop a pump with the following characteristics:

Volume flow : 3 liters/min = $5 \cdot 10^{-5}\,\text{m}^3/\text{s}$
Pressure head : 100 mmHg = $1.33 \cdot 10^4\,\text{N/m}^2$
Impeller diameter: 6 mm = $6 \cdot 10^{-3}\,\text{m}$.

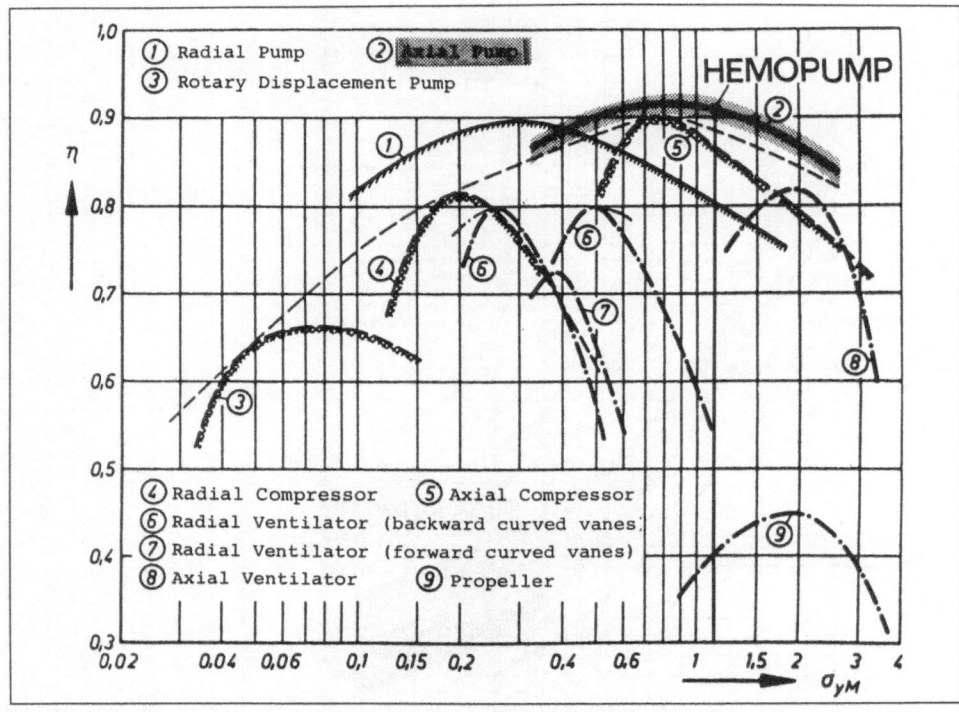

Fig. 3. Efficiency distribution as a function of specific speed for turbo machines.

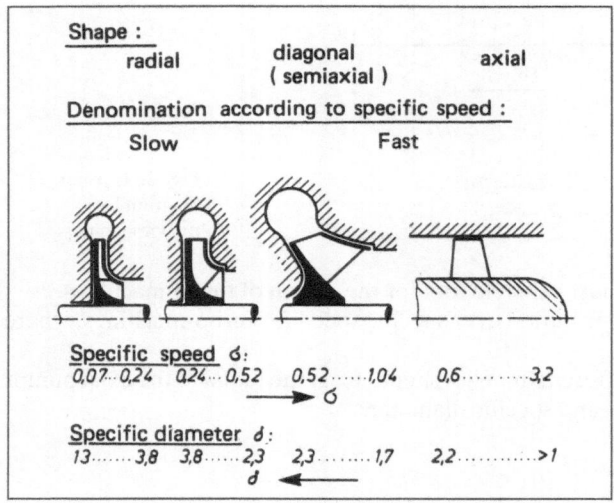

Fig. 4. Correlation of specific speed, specific diameter and impeller shapes.

From the required pressure head of $1.33 \cdot 10^4$ N/m² and the density of blood, we can calculate the specific work y (13).

Specific work:

$$y = \frac{\Delta p}{\rho} = \frac{1.33 \cdot 10^4}{1.06 \cdot 10^3} = 12.55 \frac{m^2}{s^2} \ .$$

Under the assumption that the impeller diameter should be 6 mm and the flow 3 liters/min, we can also calculate the specific diameter δ (16).
Specific diameter:

$$\delta = 1.054 \cdot D \cdot \frac{y^{1/4}}{\dot{V}^{1/2}} = 1.054 \cdot 6 \cdot 10^{-3} \cdot \frac{12.55^{1/4}}{(5 \cdot 10^{-5})^{1/2}} = 1.66 \quad .$$

With this value of δ = 1.66, we turn the Cordier diagram to the midline of the optimum efficiency range and obtain on the abscissa a value for the specific speed σ = 1.55.

We also see that we are in range 3, which is valid for axial pumps.

From the specific speed we can now calculate the necessary rotational speed of the axial pump by means of 17.

$$n = \frac{\sigma \cdot y^{3/4}}{2.108 \cdot \dot{V}^{1/2}} = \frac{1.15 \cdot 12.55^{3/4}}{2.08 \cdot (5 \cdot 10^{-5})^{1/2}} = 514 \, \text{sec}^{-1} = 30860 \, \text{min}^{-1} \quad .$$

We obtain a rotational speed of 30860 RPM. From Fig. 3 we also see that, with a specific speed of 1.15, we are in a high efficiency range of about 90% and Fig. 4 confirms that with a specific speed of 1.15 and a specific diameter of 1.66 we have to design a high speed axial pump.

Conclusions

The calculations show that the current design of the Hemopump complies with established engineering criteria for turbo-machinery and that the pump operates at a high efficiency.

If we look to the future and consider an even smaller pump with an impeller diameter of about 4 mm, but otherwise identical flow and pressure requirements, we can carry out similar calculations and obtain a minimum rotational speed of at least 54000 RPM, i.e., in the optimum efficiency range.

The first co-axial flow pump for human use: the Hemopump

R.K. Wampler

Nimbus Medical, Inc., Rancho Cordova, California, USA

History of the Hemopump

Many people ask me how I thought up this idea. It came about when I traveled to Egypt to work in a village just outside Cairo with the Bedouin people to evolve a plan to solve the problem of contaminated drinking water. During this visit I learned a piece of information that helped me design the Hemopump. Based on the principle of a submersible pump, we pumped water from a deep well. When applied to the problem of pumping blood, I thought, why not create a heart pump that pumps from inside the bloodstream?

The Hemopump is a very simple form of turbo machinery, based on the Archimedes screw. The rotor rotates at 25,000 rpm. The energy comes to the blood by the tangential velocity of the rotor. The surface speed, around 5 meters/second, is about the peak speed of blood in the aortic valves during exercise. So, we are not far from physiological speeds, and hemolysis has proven to be surprisingly low in the majority of cases.

Design

The Hemopump system includes both disposable elements and a control console. The disposable pumping system consists of an inlet cannula, an axial flow blood pump (Fig. 1), a drive cable contained in a polymeric sheath, and a motor rotor and bearing set. The inlet cannula, blood pump, and a portion of the sheath are inserted in the femoral artery and advanced through the aorta until the inlet cannula has passed retrograde through the aortic valve, with the tip positioned within the left ventricle (Fig. 2).

The Hemopump blood pump is a 21-French axial flow device with a 20-cm long inlet cannula. The blood flow through the pump is as illustrated in Fig. 2, with the tip of the inlet cannula designed for ease of insertion through the aortic valve. Blood is withdrawn from the left ventricle and discharged from the pump into the descending aorta. The pump is driven by a flexible cable that is enclosed in a 9-French sheath. The sheath also serves as a conduit for a 40% dextrose purge fluid. The fluid is used to lubricate the drive cable and hydrodynamic bearings, which support rotating elements of the device. Purge fluid flows outward through the pump seal to prevent entry of blood elements into the pumping mechanism. In the patient the drive cable exits the femoral artery and leads to the drive motor. Thus, only a 9-French diameter sheath remains within the lumen of the femoral artery. The drive motor consists of a disposable enclosed rotor attached to the drive cable, which is inserted in a nondisposable stator assembly. Purge fluid is supplied to the pump assembly by means of a roller pump, which draws fluid from a standard disposable i.v. bag.

The Hemopump controle console contains the roller pump, motor control electronics, monitor and alarm displays, and replaceable rechargeable batteries for back-up power.

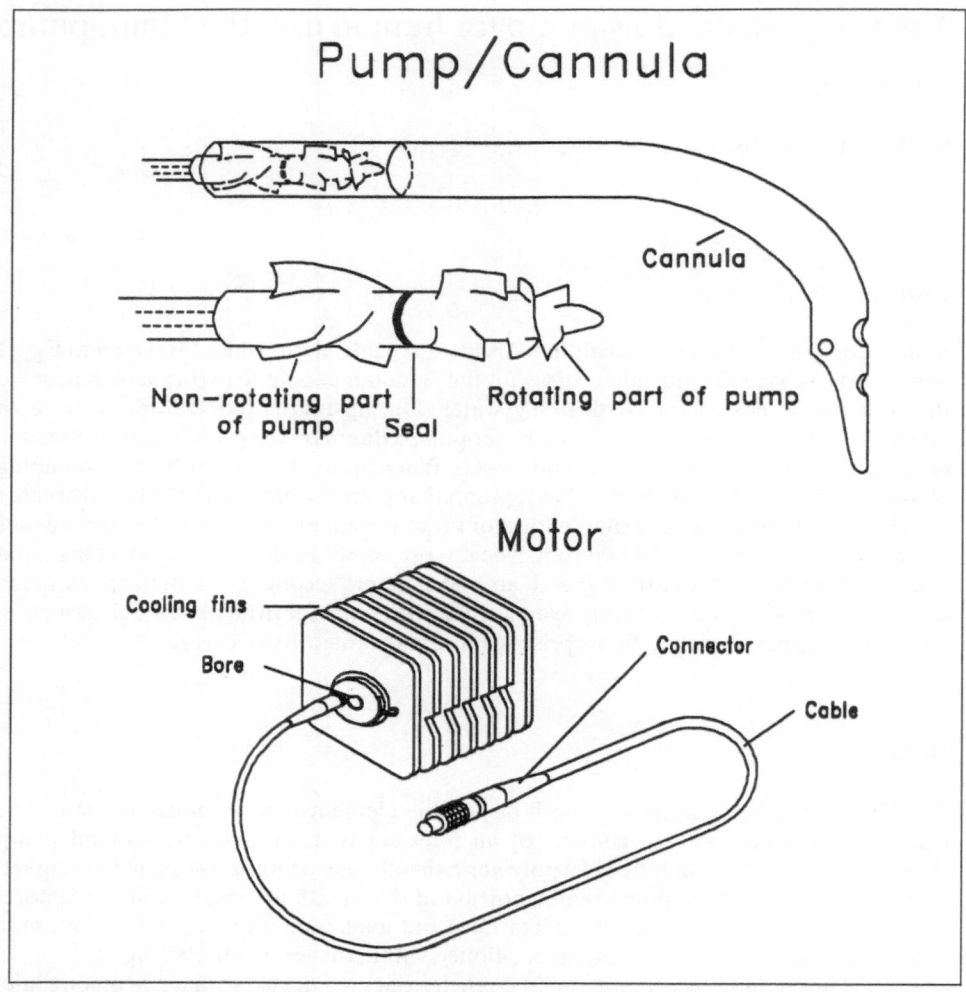

Pump/Cannula

Cannula

Non−rotating part of pump

Seal

Rotating part of pump

Motor

Cooling fins

Bore

Connector

Cable

Fig. 1. The Hemopump assembly consists of an inlet cannula, a drive cable contained in a polymeric sheath, a motor rotor and bearing set, and an axial blood flow pump.

Experience with the Hemopump in experimental animals

This is a review of some experimental work being done on the Hemopump by Dr. Richard Smalling at the Hermann Hospital, University of Texas in Houston.

Drs. Smalling and Merhige published an article in Circulation [1] which describes the effect of the Hemopump on the area at risk during acute coronary ligation in the dog. They instumented dogs with sonic micrometers in order to look at ventricular wall motion. Through left atrial catheters and arterial lines, they were able to infuse radiolabeled microspheres which were used to measure regional tissue perfusion. After creating an ischemic event, the myocardial mechanics and perfusion could be measured comparing the unassisted ventricle versus Hemopump assistance.

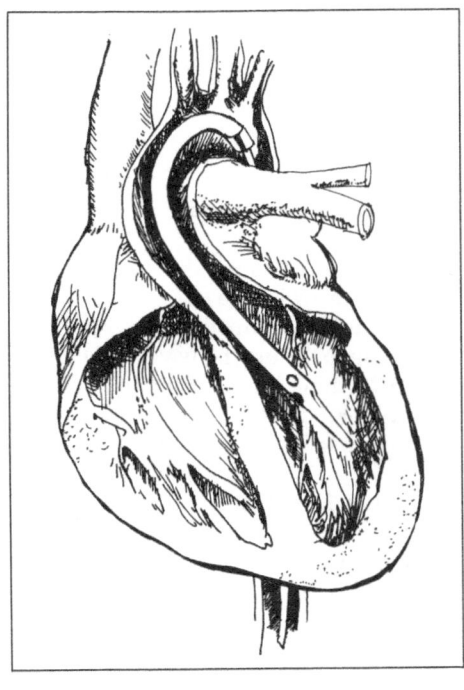

Fig. 2. The correct positionig of the pump through the femoral artery, aorta, and into the left ventricle.

While instrumented, the animals were put on the Hemopump. An ischemic event was created by occluding the left anterior descending (LAD) coronary artery. Pump on/pump off trials with and without the occlusion were performed. Then the Hemopump was left on for a total of 2 h with the LAD occluded. When the LAD occlusion was released, the Hemopump was left on for an additional 1 h.

The idea was to mimic a cardiac catheterization laboratory accident in which a coronary vessel was occluded, and to evaluate what benefit the Hemopump might provide by mechanically assisting the heart immediately after abrupt closure.

The other purpose of this study was to do a comparison of the intraaortic balloon pump (IABP) with the Hemopump in the setting of an acute occlusion.

The following results were obtained:

- The end-diastolic pressure (with Hemopump assistance) fell from a mean of about 8.1 to 3.9 mmHg (p=.005). No difference was seen with the IABP.
- There was a 30 mmHg drop in peak systolic pressure with the Hemopump, but also a drop with the IABP. There was no statistical difference noted.
- It was noted that it took 1 or 2 h for the heart to become totally unloaded while on the Hemopump. It takes time for the myocardium to realize it does not have to contract as forcefully to support the circulation.
- By the end of 2 h, we saw transient negative pressure in the left ventricle in response to Hemopump assistance
- When looking at the ischemic vs. the non-ischemic zone, we observed a predictable phenomenon. There was a shift in the regional flow balance during pump assistance. Thus, by decreasing transmural pressure and increasing the perfusion gradient combined with the auto-regulation of the coronaries, there was an increased flow into the ischemic zone, shifted from the non-ischemic myocardium.

13

– When the Hemopump was implemented within 15 min of the occlusion, we saw only a very small infarction. It appears, in comparison with the IABP, that we probably saved at least double the amount of myocardium at risk.

Initial experience in patients with acute infarction and cardiogenic shock

Infarct intervention and preservation of myocardium is not the focus of the studies we are doing in the USA now. We are, basically, looking at patients who are close to death and seeing if we can get some improved survivability for them. The future direction is to see if we can show a clear benefit to patients who are not going to die or who have a high likelihood of survival. Can we recover myocardium at risk? I think it is an exciting question. As we look at our work and the work of others regarding reperfusion injury, we believe that reperfusion in the setting of decompression can perhaps turn back time in terms of muscle injury.

Dr. Smalling has measured the ventricular pressures in humans with LV catheters during Hemopump insertion. Pressures were recorded during on/off trials. These results are not statistical, and are anecdotal at present. Here are the results in three patients with cardiogenic shock with the Hemopump in place:
– While on the Hemopump, there was a rise in the MAP from 45 to over 70. The majority of the myocardial oxygen consumption of the heart takes place during isovolumetric contraction. Thus, if you are able to reduce the peak systolic pressure and the wall radius so the wall tension is down, one can affect huge reductions in myocardial oxygen consumption.
– With the Hemopump off, the peak systolic pressure was up to 60 with an MAP of about 45.
– The Hemopump pumps more blood at lower pressures (see Fig. 3), so if the MAP is up to 100 mmHg., lower flows will be achieved. We have been giving nipride or nitroglycerine to lower the peripheral resistance to maintain mean pressures of 50–60 mmHg. This increases the pump flow and, therefore, increases cardiac output.
– The PCWP was reduced by 50% while on the Hemopump.
– Cardiac output increased more steeply after 12–24 h. The mean cardiac output rose from 2.5 to about 5.5 L/m.

In order for the Hemopump to be useful for infarct intervention, we need to design a device that is easier for the cardiologist to insert, something amenable to percutaneous insertion. Currently, a smaller size Hemopump (14F) is under development.

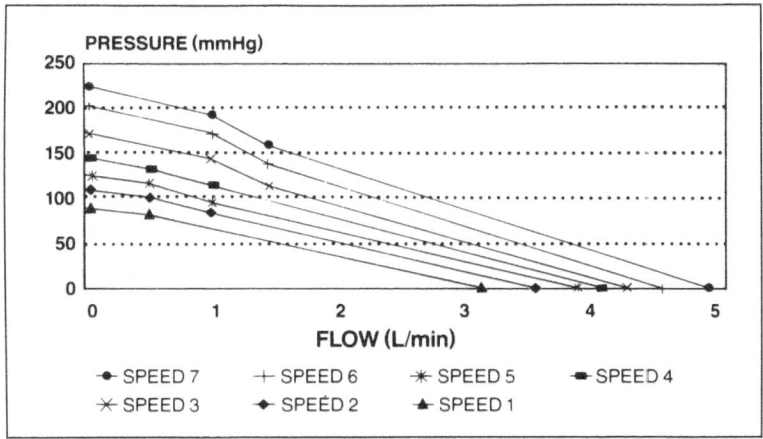

Fig. 3 Pump flow rates as a function of mean arterial pressure at each pump rate setting (in vitro testing).
The horizontal axis is pump flow rate in liters/min;
The verticle axis is pump differential pressure in mmHg.

References

1. Merhige ME, Smalling RW, Cassidy D, Barrett R, Wise G, Short J, Wampler RK: (1989) Effect of the Hemopump left ventricular assist device on regional myocardial perfusion and function. Circulation 80 (Suppl III): 158–166

Effect of the Hemopump in cardiogenic shock and in the early stage of regional myocardial ischemia

K.H. Scholz, J.P. Hering, T. Schröder, P. Uhlig, U. Tebbe, H. Kreuzer, G. Hellige

Abteilung Kardiologie und Abteilung Experimentelle Kardiologie, Georg-August-Universität Göttingen, FRG

Introduction

Currently available left-heart bypass systems are exceedingly elaborate with regard to both implantation and handling (17). Thus, in patients with cardiogenic shock, these systems are not routinely used, with the exception of occasional postcardiotomy and bridging to transplant-applications (6). Up to now, only intraaortic balloon counter-pulsation (IABP) has gained major clinical relevance in treatment of patients with cardiogenic shock (6,12). Counterpulsation leads to an improvement of cardiac energy balance, reducing left-ventricular (LV) pressure load and increasing coronary perfusion pressure. However, with this technique clinical improvement depends on residual left-ventricular function, and many patients who have ventricular failure refractory to IABP require a more complete form of mechanical support.

In contrast to IABP, the new left-ventricular assist device Hemopump (19) is capable of securing active LV assistance due to a reduction of both left-ventricular pressure and volume load. The system allows transfemoral placement, and in light of present know-ledge, it seems that the Hemopump will be able to supplement left-ventricular fuction under clinical conditions where positive hemodynamic effects can no longer be obtained with IABP.

The purpose of our studies was to assess the effects of Hemopump-left-ventricular assist on hemodynamics and myocardial energetics and metabolism in experimental cardiogenic shock, as well as during acute myocardial ischemia.

Material and methods

Conventional open-chest preparation was performed in adult sheep, weighing between 50 and 71 kg, under anesthesia with continuous infusion of buprenorphine (0.01 mg/kg*h) and midazolam (0.25 mg/kg*h) and artificial respiration (nitrous-oxide/oxygen: 70/30%).

The Hemopump was inserted via an iliac artery and placed in the left ventricle under fluoroscopic control.

The following parameters were determined and monitored (all analog data were recorded on a 10-channel recorder):

Hemodynamics: ECG; left-ventricular pressure (PLV, catheter-tip manometer); left-ventricular pressure rise (dp/dt); aortic, central venous, and pulmonary artery pressures (conventional catheters, Statham P 23 ID transducers); cardiac output (CO, thermo-dilution-technique); myocardial blood flow (Vcor, electromagnetic coronary sinus outflow-measurement (8)); myocardial perfusion pressure (difference between diastolic aortic-

and left-ventricular enddiastolic pressure); coronary, systemic and pulmonary vascular resistance.

Energetics: myocardial oxygen consumption (MVO2 = Vcor*AVDO2 (AVDO2 = arterial-coronary-venous oxygen difference)); myocardial pumping efficiency (i.e. the, percentage of the total used myocardial energy transformed in pressure-volume work: Pump. Eff. = MAP*CO*const/Vcor*AVDO2 (MAP = mean aortic pressure; CO = cardiac output)); total body oxygen consumption (TBVO2 = CO*AVDO2 (AVDO2 = arterial-central-venous oxygen difference)).

Metabolism: Release of ischemia markers (coronary venous and arterial blood samples were taken and assayed for lactate, phosphate, and potassium).

Regional myocardial wall function: epicardial electromagnetic distance transducers (7); triangle-formation of three transducers allowed on-line determination of surface areas (depending on ischemic regions during LAD-ecclusion) (9).

Experimental protocols

Studies were designed in three different parts using Hemopump in
- *cardiogenic shock*, induced by high-frequency ventricular pacing (n = 15; epicardial pacing with frequencies reducing mean aortic pressures to less than 60 mmHg in each animal).
- pacing-induced *ventricular fibrillation* (n = 9); termination by defibrillation after 30 min of fibrillation; measuring-points: at control, 10, 20, and 30 minutes of fibrillation and after 5 min of sinus rhythm without Hemopump-assist in the post-fibrillation phase).
- *regional myocardial ischemia* (n = 12; 3.5-min occlusions of the proximal LAD were performed using 3.0 to 4.5 mm PTCA balloon-catheters with and without running of the Hemopump in a randomized manner in each animal. Recovery time between occlusion was at least 60 min.

Statistics: All data are expressed as the mean ± standard deviation. The two-tailed paired *t*-test was used to assess statistical significance. Differences were considered statistically insignificant if the *p*-value exceeded 0.05.

Results

Pacing-induced shock (Fig. 1; Table 1)

Cardiac output (CO) was reduced from an average of 3.9 ± 0.9 L/min at starting conditions to 2.3 ± 1.7 L/min during pacing and was elevated up to 2.9 ± 1.2 L/min using

Table 1. Hemopump-assist in pacing induced cardiogenic shock

		Control	Shock	Shock + Hemopump
CO	(L/min)	3.9 ± 0.9	2.3 ± 1.7	2.9 ± 1.2
MAP	(mmHg)	90.2 ± 7.6	48.5 ± 7.6	67.0 ± 12.3
M.Pump.Eff.	(%)	19.1 ± 7.2	7.2 ± 4.1	18.0 ± 8.3
Lac.AVD	(mmol/L)	0.27 ± 0.16	−0.32 ± 0.72	0.24 ± 0.26

(Data are mean values ± SD. CO = cardiac output; MAP = mean aortic pressure; M.Pump.Eff. = myocardial pumping efficiency; Lac.AVD = arterial coronary-venous lactate difference)

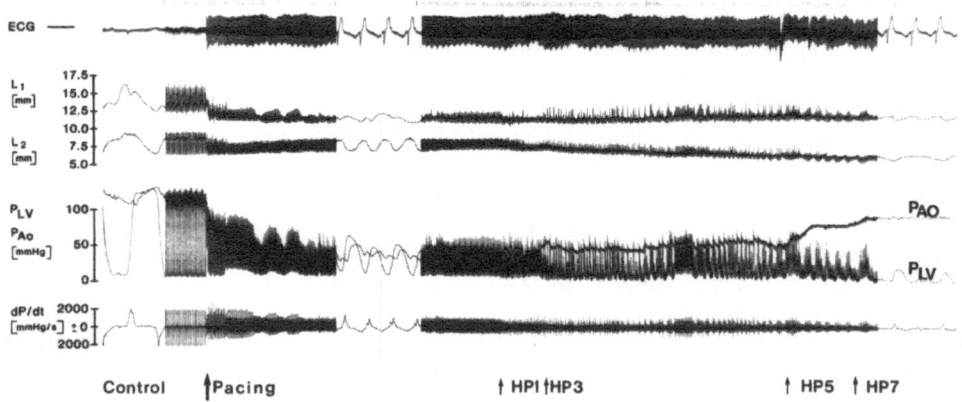

Fig. 1. Use of the Hemopump in pacing-induced shock (original record; sheep, 65 kg body weight). High-frequency pacing led to a decrease of left-ventricular systolic pressure values from 120 mmHg to about 50 mmHg. After starting the Hemopump, a gradual increase of aortic pressure (PAO) occurred, followed by a further decrease of left-ventricular pressure (PLV), registered at pump levels 1, 3, 5 and 7 (HP1–HP7). In this example mean aortic pressure at highest pump level reached about 80 mmHg.
On-line lengths measurements with epicardial distance transducers (L1; L2) showed a reduction during HP-assist, demonstrating left-ventricular unloading. (ECG: electrocardiographic; dp/dt: rate of left-ventricular pressure rise).

Hemopump at highest pump speed. Mean aortic pressures (MAP) were depressed from an average of 90.2 ± 14.5 to 48.5 ± 7.6 mmHg and elevated up to 67.0 ± 12.3 mmHg with Hemopump-assist. Coronary perfusion pressures simultaneously decreased from 65.2 to 27.3 mmHg in shock and could be significantly elevated up to 57.7 mmHg during Hemopump-assist at highest pump speed. Myocardial pumping efficiency decreased from an average of 19.1 ± 7.2% at control conditions to 7.2 ± 4.1% in cardiogenic shock and retuned to nearly normal values (18.0 ± 8.3%) during Hemopump-assist. Arterial coronary-venous lactate difference (Lact. AVD) switched from uptake (average 0.27 ± 0.16 mmol/L) to release (−0.32 ± 0.72 mmol/L) in shock and was nearly normalized (0.24 ± 0.26 mmol/L) at highest pump speed.

Ventricular fibrillation (Table 2)

Cardiac output was reduced from an average of 4.7 ± 0.8 L/min at control conditions to 2.5 ± 0.5 L/min at 10 min of fibrillation with Hemopump-assist and showed a mild

Table 2. Hemopump-assist during ventricular fibrillation

		Control	Hemopump-assist during			SR
			10'VF	20'VF	30'VF	
CO	(L/min)	4.7 ± 0.8	2.5 ± 0.5	2.4 ± 0.6	2.1 ± 0.8	2.4 ± 0.6
MAP	(mmHg)	96.8 ± 17.9	64.0 ± 14.2	60.4 ± 15.8	54.6 ± 8.1	72.2 ± 19.7
MVO2	(ml/min*100g)	9.1 ± 1.7	4.9 ± 1.5	4.9 ± 1.2	4.9 ± 1.4	6.6 ± 1.8
Pot.AVD	(mmol/L)	−0.01 ± 0.01	−0.20 ± 0.15	−0.09 ± 0.09	−0.04 ± 0.07	0.08 ± 0.37
Lac.AVD	(mmol/L)	0.32 ± 0.26	0.17 ± 0.35	0.22 ± 0.41	0.22 ± 0.37	0.28 ± 0.24

(Data are mean values ± SD. VF = ventricular fibrillation; SR = sinus rhythm, 5 min post fibrillation; CO = cardiac output; MAP = mean aortic pressure; MVO2 = myocardial oxygen consumption; Pot. AVD = arterial coronary-venous potassium difference; Lac.AVD = arterial coronary-venous lactate difference)

further decrease to 2.1 ± 0.8 L/min after 30 min of fibrillation. After defibrillation CO remained depressed for a period of time (5 min post fibrillation: 2.4 ± 0.6 L/min) in stable sinus rhythm without Hemopump-support.

Mean aortic pressure was reduced from 96.8 ± 17.9 mmHg at control to 64.0 ± 14.2 mmHg after 10 min of fibrillation with Hemopump-assist, showed a decrease to 54.6 ± 8.1 mmHg after 30 min of fibrillation and, in accordance with cardiac output remained reduced in the early phase after defibrillation (72.2 ± 19.7 mmHg).

Myocardial oxygen consumption (MVO2) decreased from 9.1 ± 1.7 ml/min*100g at control to 4.9 ± 1.5 ml/min*100g during fibrillation with Hemopump-assist and showed an increase to 6.6 ± 1.8 ml/min*100g immediately after conversion in sinus rhythm.

Arterial coronary-venous potassium difference (Pot. AVD) – being nearly zero at control-conditions – showed a significant potassium release ($-0.20 \pm .015$ mmol/L) at 10 min of ventricular fibrillation with Hemopump-assist and normalized after 30 min of fibrillation with Hemopump-support (-0.04 ± 0.07 mmol/L) (Fig. 2).

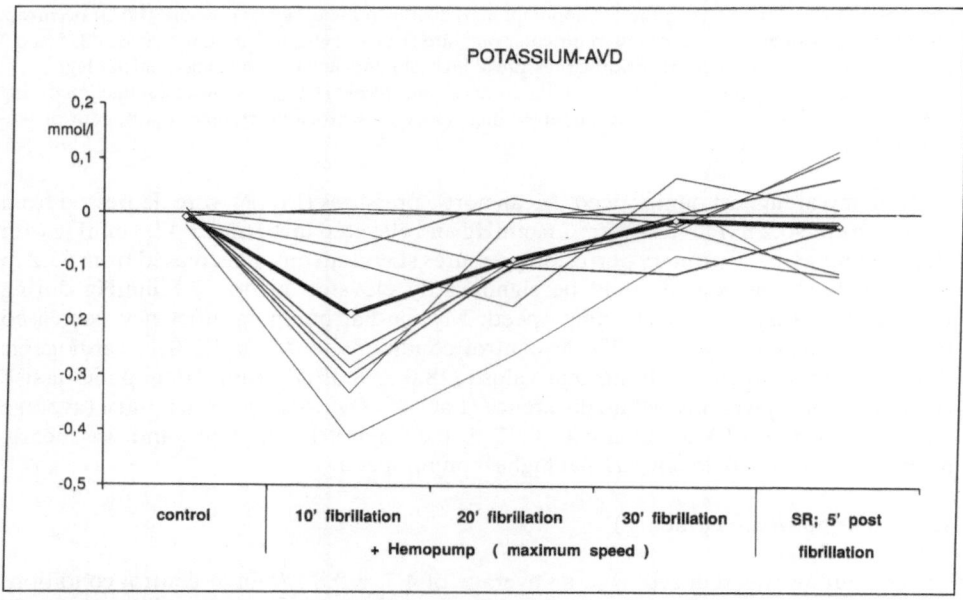

Fig. 2. Ventricular fibrillation. Graph showing arterial coronary-venous potassium difference (Pot.AVD) at control, during fibrillation and at normal sinus rhythm, 5 min after defibrillation. At normal conditions, Pot.AVD was nearly zero. In the initial period of fibrillation, we found a decrease of Pot.AVD demonstrating a marked myocardial release of potassium. In the following minutes, this potassium release was diminished and Pot.AVD normalized after 30 min of fibrillation with Hemopump-support.

Regional myocardial ischemia (Table 3)

LAD-occlusion without Hemopump-support led to ventricular fibrillation in three of 12 sheep, whereas LAD-occlusion with Hemopump-assist was followed by ventricular fibrillation in none of these animals. The data of these three animals were not considered for statistical analysis; thus, the following data result from n = 9 animals.

Table 3. Hemopump-assist in acute myocardial ischemia (LAD-Occl.)

	Pre-Occlusion		Occlusion		Reperfusion	
	without	with HP	without	with HP	without	with HP
PLVed (mmHg)	13.7 ± 4.5	9.8 ± 4.4	21.1 ± 7.2	12.1 ± 5.3	11.8 ± 1.6	9.6 ± 1.2
PAOdiast (mmHg)	72 ± 10	79 ± 11	58 ± 13	67 ± 11	59 ± 11	75 ± 5
Lac.AVD (mmol/L)	0.42 ± 0.11	0.36 ± 0.14	0.25 ± 0.22	0.42 ± 0.19	-0.50 ± 0.30	-0.19 ± 0.29
Pot.AVD (mmol/L)	-0.01 ± 0.06	0.03 ± 0.03	-0.11 ± 0.10	-0.02 ± 0.06	-0.30 ± 0.22	-0.08 ± 0.09

(Data are mean values ± SD. PLVed = left-ventricular enddiastolic pressure; PAOdiast = diastolic aortic pressure; Lac.AVD = arterial coronary-venous lactate difference; Pot. AVD = arterial coronary-venous potassium difference)

Use of Hemopump led to a significant decrease of LV enddiastolic pressure (PLVed) in the preocclusion- (from 13.7 ± 4.5 to 9.8 ± 4.4 mmHg), occlusion- (from 21.1 ± 7.2 to 12.1 ± 5.3 mmHg) and reperfusion-period (from 11.8 ± 1.6 to 9.6 ± 1.2). Due to the simultaneous increase of diastolic aortic pressures using Hemopump, we observed a significant increase of coronary perfusion pressures from 59.7 to 69.2 mmHg in the preocclusion-, from 37.0 to 54.9 mmHg in the occlusion- and from 47.2 to 65.4 mmHg in the reperfusion-period (Fig. 3).

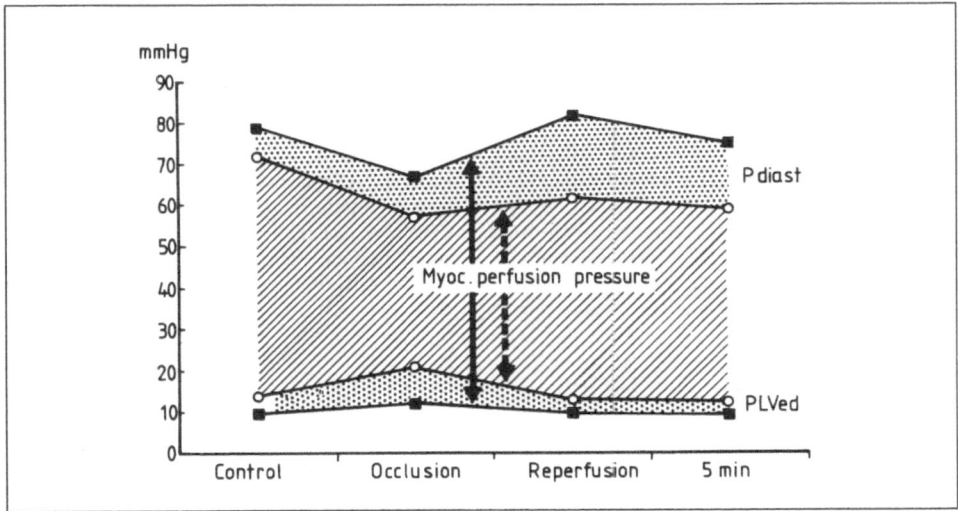

Fig. 3. Hemopump-support during LAD-occlusion. Running of the Hemopump led to both a decrease of left-ventricular enddiastolic pressures (PLVed, lower graphs) and an increase of diastolic aortic pressures (Pdiast, upper graphs) in the preocclusion-, occlusion- and reperfusion-period. This led to a marked increase of coronary perfusion pressures using Hemopump during the early stage of regional myocardial ischemia (○ = mean-values without Hemopump; ■ = mean-values with Hemopump; shaded area = perfusion-pressure without Hemopump-assist, additionally dotted area = perfusion-pressure with Hemopump-assist).

LAD-occlusion led to a marked release of lactate and potassium, mainly observed during the early reperfusion-period. Using the Hemopump during occlusion, both myocardial lactate- and potassium-release could be significantly diminished (early reperfusion-period: Lact. AVD from -0.50 ± 0.30 to -0.19 ± 0.29 mmol/L and Pot. AVD from -0.30 ± 0.22 to -0.08 ± 0.09 mmol/L during Hemopump-assist).

Analysis of regional myocardial wall function during LAD-occlusion showed a reduction of endsystolic as well as enddiastolic areas in the dependent ischemic region without changing the "bulging" phenomenon (see Fig. 4).

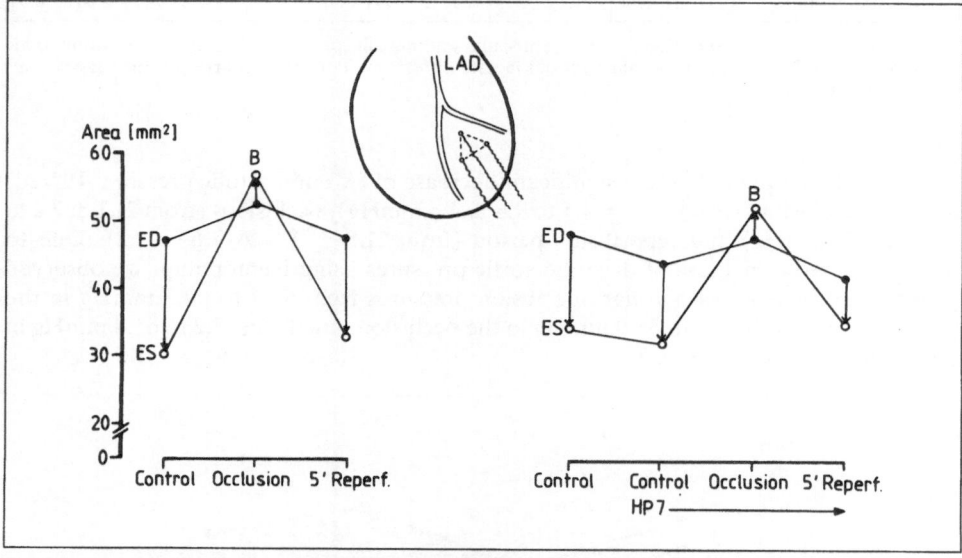

Fig. 4. Analysis of regional myocardial wall function during LAD occlusion. Epicardial electromagnetic distance transducers installed in triangle-formation at the depending ischemic region allowed on-line area calculation. At LAD occlusion, the endsystolic areas (ES, m) became larger than the enddiastolic areas (ED, l) – the systolic "bulging" phenomenon (B). Using Hemopump-support (as shown on the right side), we found a reduction of ED as well as ES, without influencing the bulging. (HP7 = Hemopump-assist at highest pump-level; all values are mean values of $n = 9$).

Discussion

Using the new Hemopump cardiac assist device in vitro, continuous blood flows of up to 4.0 liters per minute can be provided. Preliminary in vivo testings in animals revealed good anatomic compatibility, mild thrombocytopenia, and small increases in plasma-free hemoglobin, indicating only minimal hemolysis during continuous operation of up to 2 weeks (19). These findings were confirmed by initial experiences in first human use (3, 10, 13, 15).

Our data, obtained in an animal experimental model which is – with regard to body weight and hemodynamics – almost comparable to the situation in humans, demonstrate positive effects of the Hemopump both in severe cardiogenic shock, as well as in acute myocardial ischemia.

Cardiogenic shock

High-frequency ventricular pacing is followed by a depression of LV-function with a marked reduction of cardiac output and systolic left-ventricular and aortic pressures, an

22

increase of LV-enddiastolic pressures, and a decrease of myocardial perfusion pressures (1). This shock-model is reversible and reproducible and thus suitable for comparative interventional studies. Our results showed an improvement of hemodynamics using Hemopump-support (4. 16), with an increase of cardiac output and mean aortic pressures and a left-ventricular unloading indicated by a marked reduction of LV-end-diastolic pressures. This led to nearly normalized myocardial perfusion pressures in severe shock and resulted in a marked improvement of cardiac energetics and myocardial metabolism, as expressed by the increase of "pumping-efficiency" and the reversal of shock-induced myocardial release of lactate, phosphate and potassium.

Ventricular fibrillation

During ventricular fibrillation we found stabilizing effects of Hemopump-assist on hemodynamics, initially reaching cardiac output of nearly 2.5 liters per min and mean aortic pressures of more than 60 mmHg. The observed marked myocardial release of potassium was probably due to reversible damage at cellular levels and possibly caused by the initial period of high frequency pacing and the consecutive short period of fibrillation without pump support. In the further run arterial-coronary-venous potassium differences nearly normalized during Hemopump-support. Similar results were observed regarding myocardial lactate release. Myocardial oxygen consumption decreased to two-thirds of normal levels, reaching about 5 ml oxygen per min and 100 grams heart weight, which is in accordance with the known oxygen-demand of a fibrillating heart (2). These data demonstrate that the Hemopump-system should lead to sufficient oxygen supply and allows myocardial protection even at total cardiac arrest during a 30-min phase of ventricular fibrillation (14). On the other hand, in the early phase after defibrillation we found a passing left-ventricular dysfunction with a reduction in cardiac output, even though the heart was in normal sinus rhythm. These findings still indicate some reversible injury to the heart – possibly due to a myocardial catecholamine depletion – and thus further studies concerning Hemopump-assist during long term-ventricular fibrillation have to be done.

Myocardial ischemia

During LAD-occlusion, the endsystolic area of the epicardial distance-transducer formation towered over the enddiastolic area – the systolic "bulging" phenomenon (18) – indicating severe disturbances of wall motion in the dependent ischemic region. The use of Hemopump during occlusion led to a decrease of both endsystolic as well as end-diastolic areas, demonstrating left-ventricular volume unloading, but did not influence the bulging phenomenon (Fig. 4) (5). Using Hemopump during LAD-ligation in mongrel dogs, Merhige and coworkers found similar results with regard to wall motion (11). This, however, does not mean that use of Hemopump would have no beneficial effects during acute ischemia: we observed a marked increase of coronary perfusion pressures due to the decrease of LV-enddiastolic and the simultaneous increase of diastolic aortic pressures during the preocclusion, occlusion as well as the reperfusion period (4, 5). Myocardial ischemia normally leads to a marked release of lactate and potassium, most pronounced in the washing-out phase of the early reperfusion period (8). This myocardial release of lactate as well as potassium was significantly diminished in the same animals and under the same conditions during Hemopump use. We believe that, in particular, the reduction in myocardial release of potassium was responsible for the observed reduction in the incidence of ventricular fibrillation during acute ischemia. Thus, in view of these protective effects in the early stage of myocardial ischemia, Hemopump left-ventricular support could possibly be useful in different clinical situations, such as during high-risk coronary angioplasty (10).

Conclusion

Hemodynamic and metabolic data demonstrate the beneficial effects of the Hemopump, both in tachycardia-induced cardiogenic shock and ventricular fibrillation, as well as in the early stage of myocardial ischemia. According to these experimental data, the Hemopump represents a possible alternative to other heart-assist devices, as well as to intraaortic balloon counterpulsation.

References

1. Baller D, Hoeft A, Korb H, Wolpers HG, Zipfel J, Hellige G (1981) Basic physiological studies on cardiac pacing with special reference to the optimal mode and rate after cardiac surgery. Thorac Cardiovasc Surgn 29: 168–173
2. Buckberg GD, Brazier JR, Nelson RL, Goldstein SM, McConnel DH, Cooper N (1977) Studies of the effects of hypothermia on regional myocardial blood flow and metabolism during cardiopulmonary bypass 1. The adequately perfused beating, fibrillating, and arrested heart. J Thorac Cardiovasc Surg 73: 87–94
3. Frazier OH, Wampler RK, Duncan JM, Dear WE, Macris MP, Parnis SM, Fuqua JM (1990) First human use of the Hemopump, a catheter-mounted ventricular assist device. Ann Thorac Surg 49: 299–304
4. Hellige G, Uhlig P, Hering JP, Scholz KH, Schröder T, Tebbe U (1990) Effektivität des LV-Assistsystems Hemopump im kardiogenen Schock und bei regionaler Myokardischämie. Anaesthesist 39 (Suppl I): 104
5. Hering JP, Schröder T, Uhlig P, Scholz KH, Tebbe U, Hellige G (1990) Protektive Wirkung des LV-Assistsystems Hemopump in der Frühphase einer regionalen Myokardischämie. Z Kardiol 79 (Suppl I): 26
6. Kantrowitz A (1988) Circulatory support – State of the art. Trans Amer Soc Artif Intern Org 34: 445–449
7. Kebbel U, Hirche HJ (1985) An electromagnetic distance measuring system. Medical Progress through Technology 10: 213–223
8. Korb H, Hoeft A, Baller D, Wolpers HG, Hellige G, Bretschneider HJ (1984) Quantification of ischemic stress during repeated coronary artery occlusion in the dog – a method for validation of therapeutic effects. II. Reproducibility of the release and uptake of electrolytes and substrates. Basic Res Cardiol 79: 38–48
9. Korb H, Hoeft A, Böck J, Schneider A, Wolpers H, Hellige G (1986) Verbesserung der regionalen Wandfunktion im peripher- und zenralischämischen Myokard nach Hemmung der Thromboxansynthetase mit UK 38.485. Z Kardiol 75 Suppl 4: 44
10. Loisance D, Dubois Randé JL, Geschwind H, Merlet P, Deleuze PH, Lellouche D, Okude J, Castaigne A, Cachera JP (1989) Left ventricular support by intraventricular blood pump during high-risk coronary angioplasty. Lancet I: 561
11. Merhige ME, Smalling RW, Cassidy D, Barrett R, Wise G, Short J, Wampler RK (1989) Effect of the Hemopump left ventricular assist device on regional myocardial perfusion and function. Circulation 80 (Suppl 3): 158–166

12. Scholz KH, Saathoff H, Tebbe U (1989) Intraaortale Ballongegenpulsation bei akutem Myokard-infarkt, ischämischer Linksherzinsuffizienz und therapierefraktärer Angina pectoris. Dtsch med Wschr 114: 1821–1827

13. Scholz KH, Tebbe U, Chemnitius M, Kreuzer H, Schröder T, Hering HP, Uhlig P, Hellige G, Autschbach R, Dalichau H (1990) Transfemoral placement of the left ventricular assist device Hemopump during mechanical resuscitation. Thorac Cardiovasc Surgn 38: 69–72

14. Scholz KH, Schröder T, Tebbe U, Hering JP, Uhlig P, Kreuzer H, Hellige G (1990) Einsatz des linksventrikulären Assist-Systems Hemopump bei experimentellem Kammerflimmern. Z Kardiol 79 (Suppl 2): 45

15. Scholz KH, Tebbe U, Sold G, Schröder T, Hering JP, Hellige G, Autschbach R, Ruschewski W, Dalichau H, Kreuzer H (1990) Erste klinische Erfahrungen mit dem transfemoral plazierbaren linksventriculären Assist-System Hemopump. Intensivmed 27: 491–497

16. Uhlig P, Hering JP, Schröder T, Scholz KH, Ruschewski W, Tebbe U, Hellige G (1990) Protektive Wirkung des LV-Assistsystems Hemopump im kardiogenen Schock und in der Frühphase einer regionalen Myokardischämie. Thorac Cardiovasc Surgn 38 (Suppl 1): 58, 117

17. Unger F (1989) Assisted Circulation 3. Springer, Berlin, Heidelberg, New York, Tokyo

18. Vatner SF (1980) Correlation between acute reductions in myocardial blood flow and function in consciuos dogs. Circ Res 47: 201–207

19. Wampler RK, Maise JC, Frazier OH, Olsen DB (1988) In vivo evaluation of a peripheral vascular-access axial-flow blood pump. Trans Amer Soc Artif Intern Org 34: 450–455

Effects of left-ventricular assist using a co-axial flow pump (Hemopump) on organ blood flow during experimental cardiogenic shock

P. F. Wouters

University Clinic Gasthuisberg, Leuven, Belgium

Introduction

The preservation of vital organ function appears to be a critical determinant of long-term outcome in patients treated with ventricular assist devices (VAD). Renal failure and multiple organ failure are among the most frequently reported fatal complications during and following temporary mechanical circulatory assist (MCA) (14, 13). Undoubtedly, reversibility of organ dysfunction is primarily determined by the duration of cardiogenic shock which preceeds the initiation of MCA (17). However, changes in regional blood flow distribution due to the use of MCA devices may play an important role as well. Changes in hormonal and neurotransmitter tone have been reported, and it has been clearly demonstrated that MCA alters blood rheology and fluid homeostasis (5, 19). The significance of pulse pressure, the minimum perfusion pressure, and amount of flow delivered by a VAD required to maintain adequate peripheral blood flow remain to be determined. In animals with normal cardiac function, regional blood flow distribution is well maintained with the use of VAD's (6) The potential of the various types of MCA, however, to restore regional blood flow distribution following a period of critically disturbed and rapidly deteriorating regional blood flow is still controversial. Sukehiro et al. demonstrated that following a period of severe cardiogenic shock, renal blood flow could not be restored to pre-shock values with the use of a centrifugal, non-pulsatile flow VAD (18).

The Hemopump, capable of delivering up to 3.5 L/min of non-pulsatile flow has been recently classified by Mackoviak et al. as a moderate degree cardiac support system (11). Since the device can be introduced through peripheral vascular access, it combines minimal invasiveness with the efficacy of active cardiac support. For this reason, it has been stated that with the Hemopump, the application of MCA can be expanded to a larger number of patients with lesser risk (22). In order to be a good LVAD, however, the co-axial flow pump should be capable of maintain vital organ perfusion in the presence of cardiogenic shock. To address this important issue we conducted the following study: An experimental model of cardiogenic shock in dogs was developed, using a 4-h occlusion of the left anterior descending (LAD) coronary artery followed by reperfusion. MCA with the Hemopump was initiated only 90 min following myocardial ischemia and maintained for approximatively 15 h. The effects of the Hemopump on regional blood flow distribution in this model were measured using the tracer microsphere technique.

Experimental approach

Twelve mongrel dogs of either sex, weighing between 25 and 32 kg were premedicated intramuscularly with 0.25 ml/kg Hypnorm R (10 mg of fluanisone + 0.2 mg of fentanyl

27

per ml). General anesthesia was induced with 15 mg/kg sodium pentobarbital intraven-ously and maintained with a mixture of 0.5 vol% isoflurane in oxygen-enriched room air, delivered through an endotracheal tube by an Engstrom 200 respirator. Additional bolus doses of fentanyl (0.02 mg/kg) were administered intermittently when needed. Arterial blood gases were determined repeatedly throughout the experiment, and ventilation was adjusted if necessary to keep these values within the normal range.

A catheter was inserted in the right brachial artery to monitor arterial blood pressure and to obtain blood samples. A thermodilution catheter for measurement of cardiac out-put, central venous pressure, and pulmonary capillary wedge pressure was introduced through the left femoral vein. The right femoral artery was prepared for insertion of a pig-tail catheter, which could be advanced into the left ventricle for injection of tracer microspheres at appropriate times. Finally, the left carotid artery was prepared for insertion of a catheter-mounted copper coil into the LAD coronary artery (21). The position of all catheters was confirmed with fluoroscopy. Coronary artery occlusion was produced by the introduction of the copper coil (attached to a guide wire) into the LAD. The coil was positioned immediately beyond the bifurcation of the main stem. Absence of coronary perfusion distal to the coil due to an occlusive thrombus was usually achieved within 5 to 10 min and confirmed by coronary angiography with a 5F Lehman catheter. After 4 h of occlusion, the coil was withdrawn from the coronary artery, resulting in immediate reperfusion of the LAD region as confirmed again by coronary angiography. 90 min following the start of LAD occlusion, the dogs were randomly allocated either to Group 1, receiving no left ventricular assist (n=6), or Group 2, receiving Hemopump treatment until 16 h following LAD occlusion (n=6).

The Hemopump was inserted via the lower abdominal aorta through a tightly woven graft which was sutured to the vessel. The device was advanced retrogradely until its tip resided in the left ventricle. The position of the cannula was checked periodically using fluoroscopy. During pump run, heparin was administered to obtain an activated clotting time of 1.5 times the control value.

Cardiac output was determined with the thermodilution technique as the average of three successive measurements. Aortic, central venous and pulmonary artery pressure measurements were monitored through fluid-filled catheters connected to PDCR-75 Statham transducers and heart rate was calculated from the ECG tracings. Left-ventricular pressure and its first derivative (LV dp/dt) were measured using a Millar tip manometer. Estimated flow provided by the Hemopump was derived from the actual mean arterial pressure and pump speed according to in vitro calibration data of the device which are available from the Hemopump console. The pressure signals and ECG tracing were displayed on an oscilloscope and recorded on a multichannel ink jet recorder throughout the experiment.

Organ blood flow distribution was measured using the tracer microsphere technique (TM). Four differently labeled types of microspheres (15 µ diameter) were used: 141 Ce, 95 Nb, 103 Ru, and 113 Sn. Microsphere handling, dilution, and mixing was performed as described previously (3). At four different times during the experiment, the microspheres were injected through a pig-tail catheter, residing in the left ventricle: 1) during control conditions, 2) 90 min, 3) 16 h, and 4) 17 h following the start of LAD occlusion. At the end of the experiment, the organs of interest were removed and tissue samples were taken from the brain, the kidney, the liver, the small bowel, pancreas, spleen, muscle, skin, lungs, and the heart (circumflex (Cx) perfusion area, LAD perfusion area and right ventricle (RV)). The samples had an average wheight of 2 g and were placed into test tubes. Radioactivity in reference blood samples and tissue samples was counted using an automatic gamma counter and sample changer system connected to an ND 680 programmable analyzer/computer system.

Arterial blood samples were taken during control conditions and repeated 90 min, 16 and 17 h following the start of LAD occlusion. The samples were analyzed for ionic content, blood count, blood osmolality, plasma creatinine, ureum, and glycemia.

The data were analyzed using ANOVA with repeated measures (within group comparisons) and two-way ANOVA (between group comparisons). When appropriate, ANOVA was followed by Student's t-test using the modified Bonferroni correction, and alpha was set at a level of 0.05. (7) The results are presented as mean values $\pm$ SEM.

As mentioned previously, random assignment of the animals to either control or Hemopump group occurred at 90 min following the start of LAD occlusion. Prior to this event, the results of all animals were pooled and the data were analyzed accordingly. However, two-way ANOVA was performed to analyze possible between-group differences in the control conditions.

Hemodynamic outcome after Hemopump support

In the control group, five out of six animals died within 8 h following the start of LAD occlusion (Fig. 1). In this group, cardiac arrest, preceeded by a sudden decrease in cardiac output and mean arterial pressure, or ventricular fibrillation, occurred soon after the start of coronary artery reperfusion. No dog expired during the 4-h period of LAD occlusion. In the Hemopump-treated animals, all dogs survived the follow-up period of 16 h. Although in this group as well, major arrhythmias were present in almost all animals following the start of reperfusion (ventricular fibrillation in one dog, requiring electrical reconversion), total cardiac output was preserved and mean arterial pressure was maintained above 70 mmHg by Hemopump support (Table 1). Upon weaning from the ventricular assist device, one animal died in this group, and one required inotropic drug support. In four animals, however, the device could be removed without inducing major hemodynamic problems.

Mean arterial blood pressure was higher in the Hemopump-treated animals at 6 h following LAD occlusion when compared to the control group (102 ± 14 vs 49 ± 15 mmHg). In addition, the Hemopump accounted for up to 60–80% of total cardiac output. Pulmonary capillary wedge and central venous pressures did not differ between both groups.

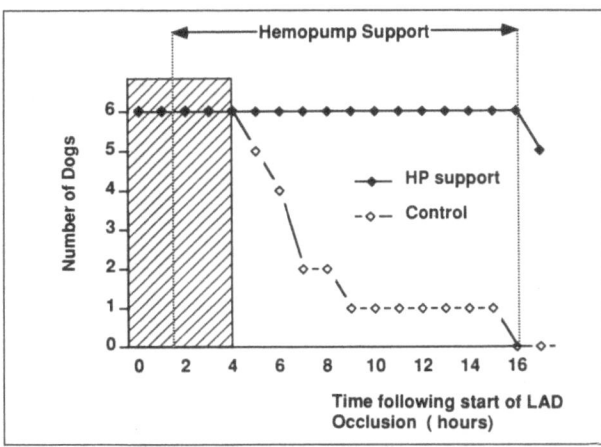

Fig. 1. Hemodynamic outcome following a 4-h occlusion with subsequent reperfusion of the left anterior descending coronary artery (LAD) in dogs with and without Hemopump support.

The shaded area indicates the 4-h period during which the LAD coronary artery was occluded.

29

Table 1. Hemodynamic performance during cardiogenic shock in untreated animals and animals treated with the Hemopump

	HR		MABP		PcWP		CVP		CO		LVSW	
	Group 1	Group 2	Group 1	Group 2	Group 1	Group 2	Group 1	Group 2	Group 1	Group 2	Group 1	Group 2
Control	85 ± 5		93 ± 5		8 ± 1		5 ± 1		4.75 ± 0.37		74 ± 3	
90 min of LAD occlusion	94 ± 9		99 ± 5		10 ± 2		5 ± 1		3.47 ± 0.27		55 ± 5*	
2 h of LAD occlusion	99 ± 8	81 ± 7	100 ± 7	96 ± 10	6 ± 3	11 ± 1	4 ± 2	5 ± 2	4.04 ± 0.68	3.55 ± 0.42	60 ± 10	59 ± 5
4 h of LAD occlusion	123 ± 15*	129 ± 23	88 ± 5	86 ± 5	7 ± 3	12 ± 2	5 ± 1	4 ± 2	5.09 ± 0.64	3.54 ± 0.71	54 ± 10*	39 ± 6*
Reperfusion	135 ± 10	110 ± 13	96 ± 12	78 ± 8	7 ± 3	13 ± 2	4 ± 2	3 ± 2	3.71 ± 0.62	2.76 ± 0.59	39 ± 8*	31 ± 8
2 h of Reperfusion	145 ± 8*	116 ± 16	102 ± 14	49 ± 15!	8 ± 4	10 ± 3	5 ± 2	4 ± 4	3.60 ± 0.48	3.02 ± 1.46	36 ± 6*	28 ± 19
16 h following LAD occlusion	174 ± 8*	–	75 ± 12	–	6 ± 3	–	4 ± 2	–	4.62 ± 0.32	–	28 ± 4*	–
1 h after HP stop	165 ± 13*	–	80 ± 11	–	8 ± 6	–	5 ± 2	–	3.44 ± 0.48	–	24 ± 5*	–

HR = Herat Rate in bpm; MABP = Mean Arterial Blood Presure in mmHg; PcWP = Pulmonary capillary Wedge Pressure in mmHg; CVP = Central Venous Pressure in mmHg; CO = Cardiac output in Liter per minute; LVSW = Left Ventricular Stroke Work in g. m. m^{-2}

Group 1: Animals treated with the Hemopump
Group 2: Untreated animals
* = $p < 0.05$ vs control, ! = $p < 0.05$ vs group 2

Regional blood flow distribution during and after Hemopump support

The presence of 90 min of LAD occlusion was reflected in a significant decrease in flow to the LAD-perfused area (Fig. 2). No other changes in regional blood flow distribution due to 90 min of coronary artery occlusion were noted.

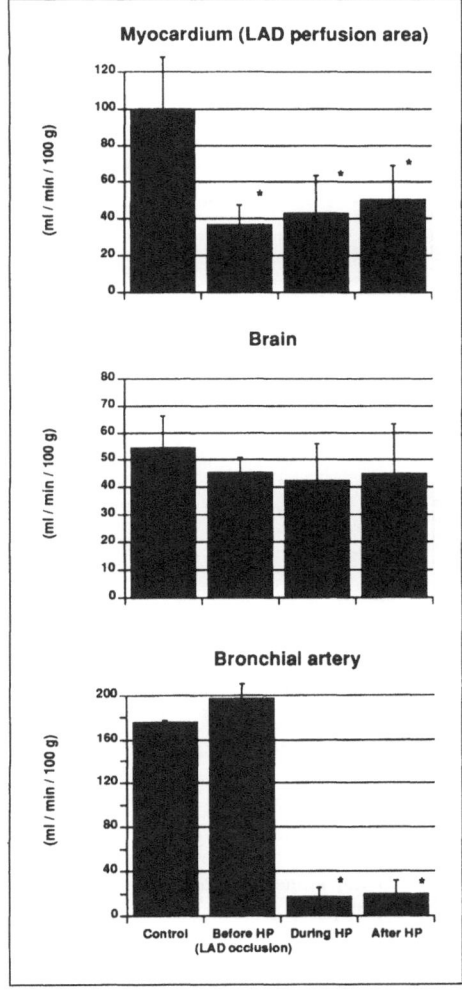

Fig. 2. Blood flow to the heart, brain and bronchi before, during and after Hemopump (HP) support. "Control" and "Before HP" represent mean ± SEM values of all experiments before randomization. "During HP" and "After HP" represent mean ± SEM values in animals treated with the Hemopump. At these intervals all untreated animals had expired.
* = p < 0.05 vs control
"During HP" reflects regional blood flow during Hemopump run in animals supported for 14.5 h. "After HP" represents flow as measured 1 h after removal of the Hemopump.
"LAD perfusion area" represents flow to the perfusion area of the temporarily occluded coronary artery.

After 14.5 h of Hemopump support, blood flow to the brain was not different from control conditions. Similarly, blood flow to the medullary and cortical area of the kidneys (Fig. 3), to the pancreas, small bowel, and spleen (Fig. 4), and to muscle and skin remained within control levels. Hepatic arterial blood flow increased (see Fig. 4) and bronchial flow decreased significantly (see Fig. 2) when compared to control. Bronchial flow remained low after withdrawal of Hemopump support. Subepicardial, but not subendocardial blood flow to the LAD perfused area restored to normal levels after reperfusion and Hemopump support. No changes were observed in blood flow to the circumflex-perfused area or the right ventricle throughout the study.

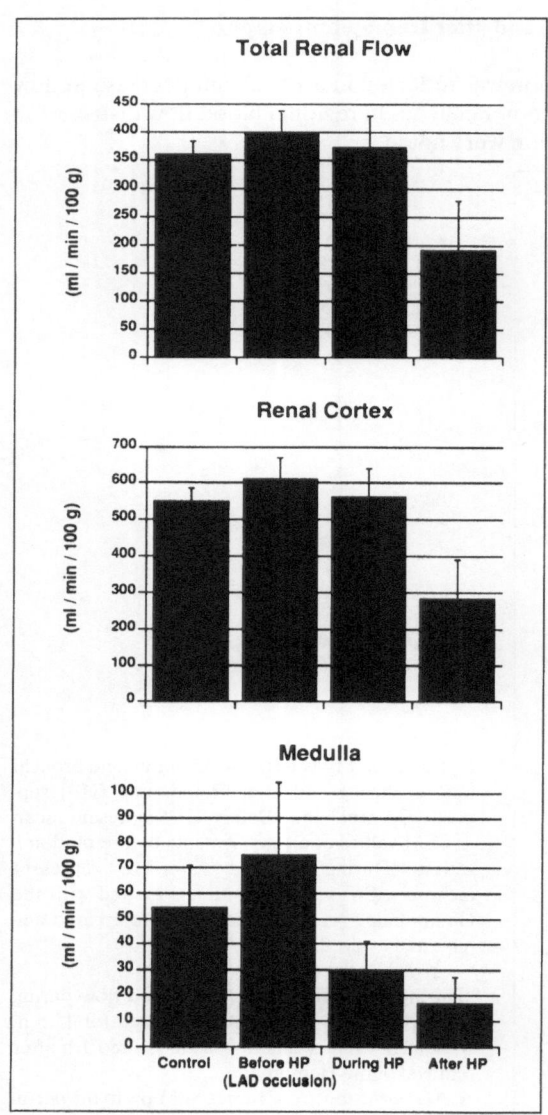

Fig. 3. Regional blood flow distribution to the kidney before, during, and after Hemopump (HP) support. (For abbreviations see Fig. 2.)

Blood analysis

After 14.5 h of Hemopump run, creatinine and BUN were maintained at control levels (creatinine: 1.3 ± 0.4 vs 0.7 ± 0.1 mg/dl at control and BUN: 35 ± 6 vs 35 ± 3 mg/dl at control). Ionic plasma content of sodium, potassium, chloride, calcium, and blood glucose remained stable throughout the study.

Platelets decreased significantly after 14.5 h of Hemopump support (from 131 ± 10 to 34 ± 12.10^3 per milliliter). Due to some continuous blood loss at the site of the Hemopump insertion, a small but not statistically significant drop in hemoglobin was noted (from 10.9 ± 1.1 to 7.9 ± 2.2 mg/dl)

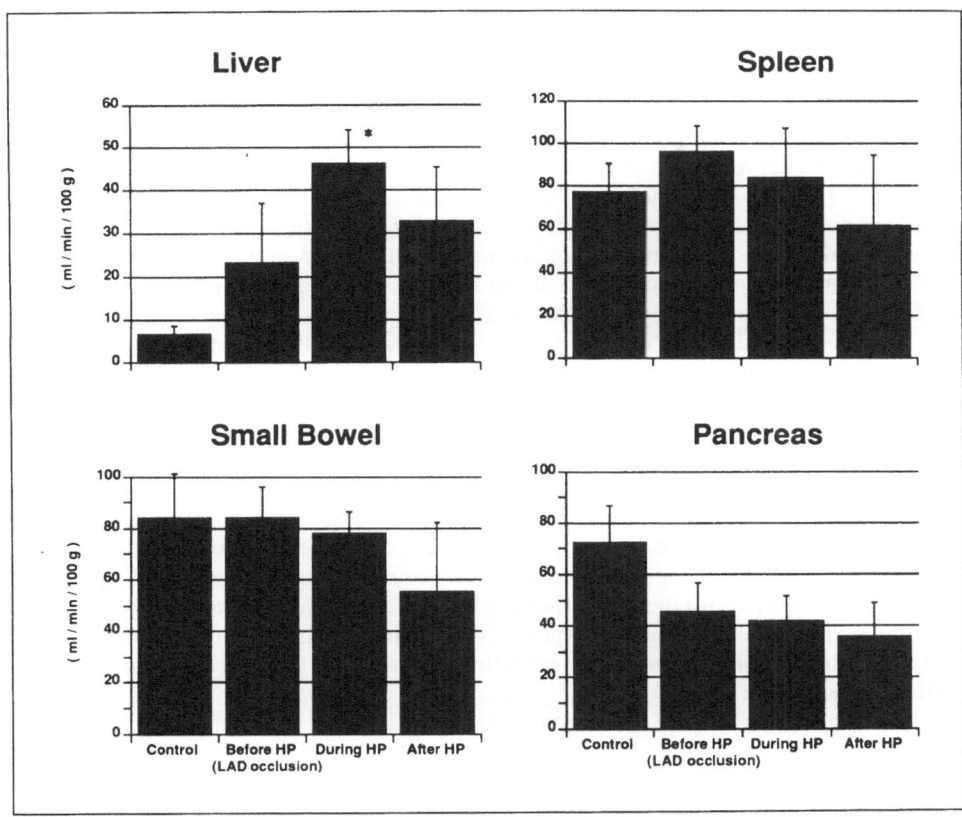

Fig. 4. Blood flow to the intestinal organs before, during, and after Hemopump (HP) support. (For abbreviations see Fig. 2.)

Discussion

Our experimental model of cardiogenic shock is very severe and shows a mortality of 100% in the control group. All Hemopump-treated animals survived the experiment, and four out of six animals were easily weaned from the LVAD, indicating that some degree of ventricular recovery had occurred. In two animals however, pump-dependency had developed and the animals required resuscitation upon weaning from the device. For these animals, the time required to recover from ischemia probably exceeded the duration of this experiment and weaning from the Hemopump was premature. It was demonstrated earlier that the time to recovery from myocardial stunning may range from several hours to days (10, 1). Nevertheless, the Hemopump appeared to adequately support global hemodynamic function and to prevent the lethal consequences of acute myocardial ischemia and reperfusion during the experiment.

The artificial maintenance of circulation by means of ventricular assist devices is of clinical value only when organ perfusion is preserved. The principle issue of this study therefore was to assess the adequacy of regional blood flow distribution during

33

Hemopump support. In all animals, resuscitated with the Hemopump for at least 14.5 h, blood flow to the kidneys, brain, muscle, skin, spleen, intestines, and pancreas were preserved. Biochemical analyses show that markers for kidney function such as plasma creatinine and ureum also remain within control values. The increase in hepatic arterial blood flow during Hemopump support might well reflect a physiologic response to a concommittant decrease in portal blood flow, generally referred to as hepatic blood flow reciprocity (16). Unfortunately, our experimental set-up did not allow us to measure portal venous blood flow. However, all measured abdominal organ blood flows contributing to portal venous flow, including pancreatic, splenic and intestinal flow decreased, although not statistically significant, during Hemopump support. Hepatic oxygen delivery is primarily influenced by changes in arterial blood flow (4). Since arterial hepatic blood flow increased during Hemopump support it is unlikely that hepatic oxygen delivery was disturbed during this period.

Bronchial arterial blood flow decreased tremendously after 14.5 h of Hemopump support. As this flow remained low 1 h after withdrawal of Hemopump support, a time-dependent factor rather than a Hemopump-induced effect may explain this finding. Alternatively, the location of the outlet cannula in the vicinity of the origin of bronchial arteries theoretically predisposes to a specific flow reduction in this area due to turbulence of flow or a Venturi-like effect. Tissue edema, atelectasis, bleeding around the bronchial arteries and collapse of the pulmonary veins due to drainage of the left atrium have been associated with the use of LVAD's (17, 18). In addition, Sukehiro et al reported an increase in alveolar to arterial oxygen difference in animals supported with an LVAD (18). The clinical implications of these findings are undoubtedly important and require further investigation.

After reperfusion of the LAD coronary artery and an extended period of Hemopump support, blood flow to the subendocardium did not restore to preocclusion values, whereas subepicardial blood flow did. Mild reperfusion abnormalities (zones of "low reflow") have been demonstrated earlier in postischemic viable myocardial tissue adjacent to an infarcted area. In addition, Vanhaecke et al. have demonstrated a reduced flow reserve in these areas of the myocardium which persists for at least 24 h following reperfusion and is possibly mediated through a reduction of adenosine availability (20). Alternatively, it can be postulated that reduced flow in the peri-infarction area results from lowered metabolic requirements in a stunned myocardium. Regardless of the cause of flow reduction in reperfused post-ischemic subendocardium, the Hemopump does not appear to influence this phenomenon. In our study, tissue samples for determination of blood flow were obtained transmurally from viable myocardium immediately adjacent to the infarct. In these samples, the subendocardium, which is more vulnerable to ischemia when compared to the subepicardium, may consist of "low reflow" areas.

Blood flow to the right ventricle was well maintained during Hemopump support. Perfusion of the non-ischemic area of the left ventricle (circumflex coronary artery perfusion area) was unaffected by Hemopump run. However, Merhige et al. showed that during coronary artery occlusion, the Hemopump caused a redistribution of coronary artery flow in favor of the ischemic area (12). For this reason and because VAD's are generally believed to reduce myocardial oxygen demand, we had expected a Hemopump-induced reduction in flow to the circumflex coronary artery perfusion area. Our findings suggest a disruption of coronary artery autoregulation resulting in inappropriately high flows to the non-ischemic area during the Hemopump. The moderate degree of support to the left ventricle as delivered by the Hemopump may be inadequate to completely unload the left ventricle. In that case, the non-ischemic area of the left ventricle is required to compensate for the decreased performance of the postischemic stunned area, thus demanding more oxygen then predicted by general LV hemodynamic indices. An alternative explanation is suggested by the findings of Dennis et al. who demonstrated that reduction of oxygen utilization by left-heart bypass is merely reflected in a reduction in arteriovenous oxygen difference rather than flow (2). Unfortunately, our preparation did not allow us to measure oxygen consumption of the heart. Finally it should be considered that Kresh et al. has shown that reduction of myocardial oxygen consumption by left heart bypass may not be as large as previously thought. Intramural pressures in the myocardium are reduced only up to 20% of pre-bypass values and are only slightly affected by the degree of cardiac unloading which can be obtained with VAD's (9).

Conclusion

In this study the Hemopump was demonstrated to adequately support global hemodynamics in a canine model of severe cardiogenic shock. Lethal hemodynamic consequences of myocardial ischemia and reperfusion were present in all untreated animals, but were prevented adequately with the use of the Hemopump. Most importantly, regional blood flow distribution was minimally affected during Hemopump support. Vital organs such as the kidney, the brain, the intestines, and the liver received adequate blood flow. Controversies with regard to myocardial perfusion remain, however, and further studies are required to elucidate the complex interaction of left-ventricular performance and myocardial oxygen balance in the presence of MCA provided by the Hemopump. In conclusion, our data suggest that the Hemopump provides safe and effective MCA in the presence of cardiogenic shock.

References

1. Bush LR, Buja LM, Samowitz W, Rude RE, Wathen M, Tilton GD, Willerson JT (1983 Recovery of Left ventricular segmental function after long-term reperfusion following temporary coronary occlusion in conscious dogs. Circ Res 53: 248–263
2. Dennis C, Hall DP, Moreno JR, Senning A (1962) Reduction of the oxygen utilization of the heart by left heart bypass. Circ Research 10: 298–305
3. Flameng W, Winkler B, Wuesten B, Schaper W (1977) Minimum requirements for the measurement of regional myocardial blood flow using tracer microspheres. Bibl Anat 15: 24–29
4. Greenway CV, Stark RD (1971) Hepatic vascular bed. Physiol Rev 51: 23–65
5. Hung T-C, Butter DB, Kormos RL, Sun Z, Borovetz HS, Griffith BP, Yie C-L (1989) Characteristics of blood rheology in patients during novacor left ventricular system support. ASAIO Transactions 35: 611–613
6. Johnston GG, Hammill F, Marzec U (1976) Prolonged pulseless perfusion in unanaesthetized calves. Arch Surg 111: 1225–1230
7. Keppel G (1982) Correction for multiple comparisons. Design and Analysis. Prentice-Hall 144–166
8. Kobayashi S, Takahashi H, Nishiyama H, et al (1982) Studies on left ventricular bypass: the preventive measure of excess negative pressure upon the inside of left atrium during left ventricular bypass. Jpn J Artif Organs 11: 131–134

9. Kresh JY, Kerkhof PLM, Goldman SM, Brockman SK (1986) Heart-Mechanical assist device interaction. ASAIO Trans 32: 437–443
10. Lavallee M, Cox D, Patrick TA, Vatner SF (1983) Salvage of myocardial function by coronary artery reperfusion 1, 2, and 3 hours after occlusion in conscious dogs. Circ Res 53: 235–247
11. Mackoviack JA, Dasse KA, Poirier VL (1990) Mechanical cardiac assistance and replacement. Heart Transplantation 8: 39–53
12. Merhige ME, Smalling RW, Cassidy D, Barret R, Wise G, Short J, Wampler RK (1989) Effect of the Hemopump Left Ventricular Assist Device on Regional Myocardial Perfusion and Function. Circulation 80 (Suppl III): III-158–III-166
13. Parascandola SA, Pae WE, Davis PK, Miller CA, Pierce WS, Waldhausen JA (1988) Determinants of survival in patients with ventricular assist devices. ASAIO Transactions 34: 222–228
14. Pennington DG, Kanter KR, McBride LR, Kaiser GC, Barner HB, Miller LW, Naunheim KS, Fiore AC, Willman V (1988) Seven years' experience with the Pierce-Donachy ventricular assist device. J Thorac Cardiovasc Surg 96: 901–911
15. Phang P T, Keough K M (1986) Inhibition of pulmonary Surfactant by plasma from normal adults and from patients having cardiopulmonary bypass. J Thorac Cardiovasc Surg 91: 248–251
16. Richardson PID, Withrington PG (1981) Liver blood flow. Gastroenterology 81: 159–173
17. Schoen FJ, Palmer DC, Bernhard WF, Pennington DG, Haudenschild CC, Ratliff NB, Berger RL, Golding LR, Watson JT (1986) Clinical temporary ventricular assist. Pathologic findings and their implications in a multi-institutional study of 41 patients. J Thorac Cardiovasc Surg 92: 1071–1081
18. Sukehiro S, Flameng W (1990) Effects of Left Ventricular Assist for cardiogenic shock on Cardiac function and Organ blood flow distribution. Ann Thorac Surg 50: 374–383
19. Taenaka Y, Yagura A, Takano H, Matsuda T, Noda H, Kinoshita M, Takatani S, Akutsu T (1988) Altered humoral control of circulating volume during artificial circulation. ASAIO Transactions 34: 692–695
20. Vanhaecke J, Flameng W, Borgers M, Jang I, Van de Werf F, De Geest H (1990) Evidence for decreased coronary flow reserve in viable postischemic myocardium. Circulation Research 67
21. Van de Werf F, Vanhaecke J, Jang I-K, Flameng W, Collen D, De Geest H (1987) Reduction in infarct size and enhanced recovery of systolic function after coronary thrombolysis with tissue-type plasminogen activator combined with β-adrenergic blockade with metoprolol. Circulation 75 (4): 830–836
22. Wampler RK, Moise JC, Frazier OH, Olsen DB (1988) In vivo evaluation of a peripheral vascular access axial flow blood pump. ASAIO Transactions 34: 450–454

II. Clinical Aspects

Investigational trials of the Hemopump

R.K. Wampler

Nimbus Medical, Inc., Rancho Cordova, California, USA

The evolution of the Hemopump

From conception to production to clinical use is a lengthy and expensive process. Over 10 million dollars have been spent on this project.

Currently, the Hemopump is 21F in size. A smaller version of the device, 14F, is being evaluated.

The console has gone through a process of evolution and is now user-friendly and reliable. It can be mounted at the foot of the bed or on a metal stand (Fig. 1). Nurses who manage this pump say it is very user-friendly in the clinical environment. They do not spend a lot of time managing the Hemopump console. Therefore, they are able to spend their time taking care of the patient. No extra people are needed at the bedside as with the Biomedicus, Centromed pumps or other LVAD.

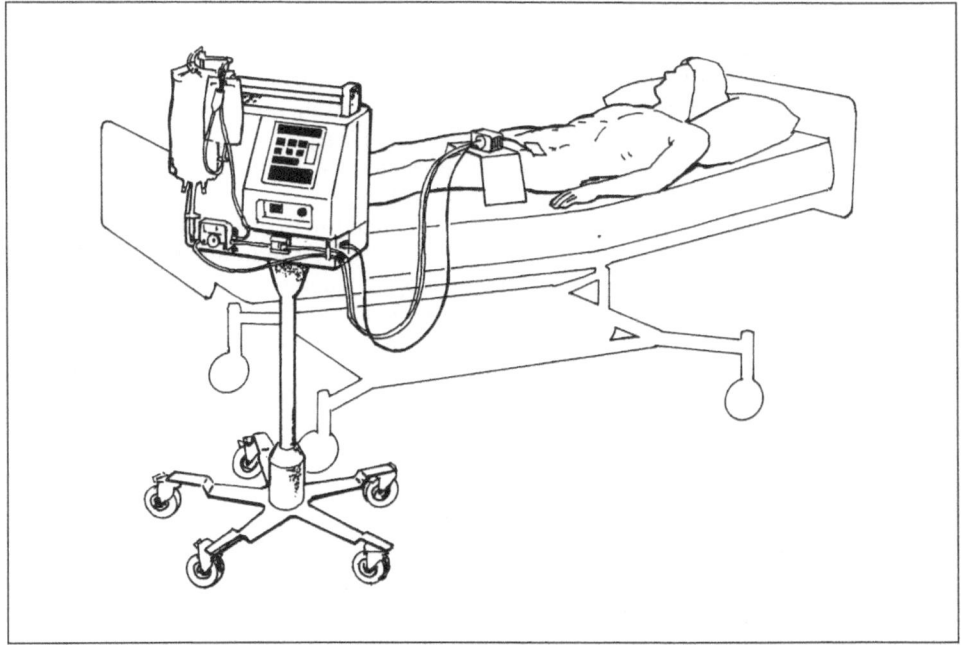

Fig. 1. The Hemopump system in the clinical setting. The indwelling pump/cannula device is inserted via the femoral artery. The flexible drive shaft is coupled to a magnet in the motor stator outside the patient's body. The power supply for the motor and control and diagnostic/alarm systems are incorporated in a portable, mobile console mounted on the foot of the patient's bed.

Hemopump clinical trials

Clinical trials are on-going at 10 centers throughout the U.S. The initial trials were designed for patients who were expected to die and had nothing to lose. Originally, the Hemopump was considered to be a radical device. The FDA permitted us to use it only with patients who had no other possible modality for treatment. We selected patients in cardiogenic shock with a reported mortality of over 80%.

Inclusion criteria

Our definition of cardiogenic shock was:
– a cardiac index (CI) of $< 2Lpm/m^2$;
– pulmonary capillary wedge pressure (PCWP) of $> 18mmHg$;
– systolic blood pressure of $< 90mmHg$.

Patients also needed to be refractory to volume therapy and pharmacological support. It was *not* a prerequisite that they failed on the intraaortic balloon pump (IABP), but 75% had.

Diagnostic etiologies

These included:
– acute myocardial infarction (AMI);
– failure to wean from cardiopulmonary bypass (CPB);
– low cardiac output syndrome following weaning from CPB;
– rejection of heart transplant.

The data presented later demonstrate that the failure to wean group had the best prognosis; low cardiac output had the worst. A very important observation was that delay in treatment is associated with very poor results. There is a point in the shock continuum where recovery of the patient is not possible. To achieve high survival, it is important to be comfortable with using this device in a timely fashion.

This is an overview of the first 53 patients evaluated for inclusion in the Hemopump study. The patients had a mean age of 54 years. They were predominantly male. There were 17 with AMI, 17 with PCS (post cariotomy support), and seven in the other category. Of the 53 that were accepted, 41 underwent successful insertion. The majority of failed insertions were failures at the iliac level or at the bifurcation of the aorta. There were a couple of patients where the device could not be negotiated around the arch. Women had a much lower success rate than men. Of those that received the device, 15/42 (35%) were successfully weaned from support and 13/42 (30%) were 30-day survivors. An additional two patients died after the 30-day follow-up period.

Many clinicians are concerned about the effect of this device on the red blood cells. Many think of this device as a "Waring blender" for red cells. It actually turns out to be relatively atraumatic to red blood cells. The non-surgical group in our study had a mean plasma free hemoglobin level of 18 mg%. The surgery group had a level of about double that amount (37 mg%). We believe the difference to be the result of roller pump support during surgery and massive blood transfusions. In general, following CPB, even with elevated levels, it was noted that the plasma free hemoglobin came down during Hemopump assistance. Large numbers of transfused units of banked blood will also raise the levels somewhat, but in general, I do not believe that the elevation is clinically significant in terms of renal injury, in the great majority of cases.

Platelets are significantly affected. Thrombocytopenia often occurs; usually, this does not require intervention and has not been associated with spontaneous bleeding. A reduction in platelets during pump operation occurs, which rises rapidly after pump removal. This is not too different from the thrombocytopenia seen during use of the intraaortic balloon pump (IABP).

Safety

We sought to get a post-mortem examination on all patients who died, and we also performed echocardiography follow-up on survivors to 30 days. We have seen one patient that had a small fenestration of the aortic valve at post-mortem exam. This was not thought to be hemodynamically significant, but was recorded as a device-related complication. We have not seen clinical or echocardiographic evidence of significant aortic insufficiency. We have not seen injury to papillary muscles or to intracardiac structures. The degree of intravascular hemolysis observed during Hemopump support is negligible in most cases, and has not been implicated as a cause of patient injury or death.

Complications

We have seen some cases of arterial injury related to trauma during pump insertion. These have been repaired either with grafts or with vein patches, and to date there has *not* been a reported episode of leg ischemia. We have seen two cases of cerebral vascular accident. Both of these cases occurred after pump removal, 1 week to 18 days afterward. One was associated with a pre-Hemopump mural thrombus in an AMI patient, and the other was associated with atrial fibrillation and a mural thrombus. We have seen significant bleeding in some of the surgery cases, and some significant bleeding associated with the administration of streptokinase or TpA in the AMI patients.

Case examples

Case 1: The first AMI patient we did was a 33-year old woman in Michigan who thought herself to be in good health until she developed some symptoms she associated with indigestion. She waited a day before seeing her physician. By the time she was seen, she had developed significant shock and was admitted to the hospital. She underwent angiography during which she developed some episodes of ventricular fibrillation. In response to this, she was started on the intraaortic balloon pump and was followed for about 5 days, after which she was transferred to the University of Michigan. It was recognized that she was in a terminal condition. She was placed on the Hemopump and in response developed a very rapid hemodynamic response and subsequent left-ventricular recovery. She was discharged about 2 weeks from the time of her admission.

Case 2: This patient was experiencing a very rapid sinus tachycardia prior to the Hemopump insertion. It resolved after the pump was placed. In general, I would expect to see some reduction in tachycardia in response to Hemopump assistance, but this response was much more dramatic than is typically observed.

One thing that surprised us and other investigators was that the total cardiac output in most patients does not typically change in the immediate post-insertion period. More commonly, a shift of the work burden from the left ventricle to the Hemopump is seen. So, a patient with a cardiac output of 3.5 L/min. may have an output of 3.5 to 4 L/min. after 12 h. One difference will be a reduction in the pulse amplitude between systole and diastole. The pulse amplitude will narrow significantly if good assistance is achieved. Ideally, it will be possible to stop many of the drugs given to maintain the cardiac output.

Pulmonary capillary wedge pressure (PCWP) might be expected to fall rapidly and does. If a patient on the Hemopump does not show a significant reduction in the PCWP, we would be very suspicious that something is wrong. Perhaps the pump is not positioned properly, has been damaged during insertion or has aspirated a mural thrombus. Another possible problem could be that the patient has a septal defect (shunting) or an incompetent valve. One should observe a significant decompression of the left atrium, even if the cardiac output does not go up and even if a rise in mean arterial pressure does not follow pump insertion.

The pulse amplitude is a very good way of tracking efficacy and insures that the patient is, indeed, being assisted. It is very important to watch this parameter during Hemopump assistance. The pump does *not* have a feedback mechanism that confirms that it is pumping across the valve. The nurses or other support personnel, who are watching the patient, must be aware of the clinical parameters that confirm good assistance. One of these is a decreased pulse width and the other is to watch the patient for any sudden changes. It is possible for a patient to throw a mural thrombus and obsctruct the pump. It is also possible for a cannula to be ejected from the ventricle. In pumpdependent patients this may be catastrophic.

Case 3: This patient started out with an ejection fraction of about 16% which doubled at the time of pump removal. The patient had a massive anterior infarction and lost a lot of septum. I don not believe we were able to save any of her heart muscle because of the delay in treatment. But, we did save her life and she is functional. She is able to do her activities, some walking and is quite happy with her lifestyle.

The goal of mechanical assistance is to perfuse the circulation and decrease the work of the left ventricle. Fortunately, we are dealing with a very steep part of the curve in terms of the Starling curve and LaPlace's law. So, a small reduction in pre and afterload of the heart by reducing the left-ventricular pressure will be associated with a marked improvement in pulmonary edema and a marked improvement in contractility and increased perfusion of ischemic myocardium.

We would like to stress the importance of proper placement of the Hemopump. The drive cable has stress concentration when placed too high in the aortic arch. It can be fractured if it is bent too much during operation. If the pump gets too high into the arch or is traumatized during insertion, fracture may occur and the Hemopump will have to be removed and replaced with a new one. If a blind insertion is necessary, a follow-up x-ray should be taken immediately to be sure the pump housing is down in the descending arch. Placement under fluoroscopy is recommended, however.

Efficacy and control study

We performed a study comparing the results of the Hemopump with those of the IABP. One objective of this analysis was to define which patients are most appropriate candidates for Hemopump insertion. In my opinion, the biggest mistake is waiting too long to use the Hemopump. Bill Pierce in the USA, who works with artificial hearts, states "You know, these wonderful mechanical devices can support life but they cannot create life". If the Hemopump becomes the kind of device that is used in desparation after the failure of all conventional treatment, the results are going to be very discouraging. If the device is used at a time when there is *not* multiple organ failure and irreversible shock, results can be very good.

We did a retrospective study of patients on the IABP for a control. We pulled patient records sequentially on patients that met the diagnostic criteria of shock and had received the IABP at the investigation institutions. We quickly discovered that there were not many patients that met our criteria. There are very few patients with a cardiac index of < 2, a PCWP > 18, and hypotension. We stratified the patients by single hemodynamic parameters to try to find common elements.

Patients with an elevated PCWP (> 20 mmHg) at the time of IABP insertion had a fairly high mortality (see Fig. 2). So, we stratified this group with the Hemopump group which had a PCWP of > 20 mmHg. Although this is not statistical, we saw three times the number of survivors in Hemopump patients compared to IABP patients (37% vs. 13%). We saw one survivor with a PCWP of 30 mmHg, this is very unusual. Whenever a patient 's PCWP reaches 30–35 mmHG., they are very far along in shock and it is difficult to reverse the process.

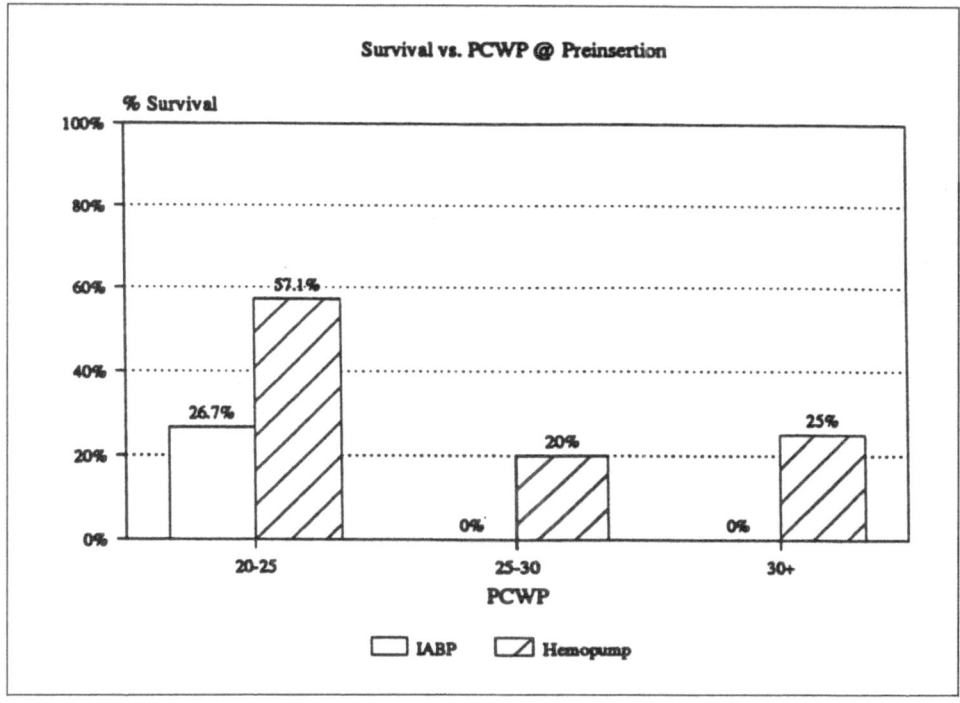

Fig. 2. Relationship between survival of patients treated with IABP or Hemopump and pre-insertion pulmonary capillary wedge pressure (PCWP expressed in mmHg).

We found the cardiac index to be a bit better as a discriminator (see Fig. 3). We compared the IABP patients and the Hemopump patients who had a cardiac index of < 2 Lpm/m^2 for 30-day survival. We found that 7% of the IABP survived, versus 32% survival for the Hemopump patients. The *p* value of this group was statistically not significant. When the cardiac index is below 1.5 Lpm/m^2, it is difficult to achieve survival.

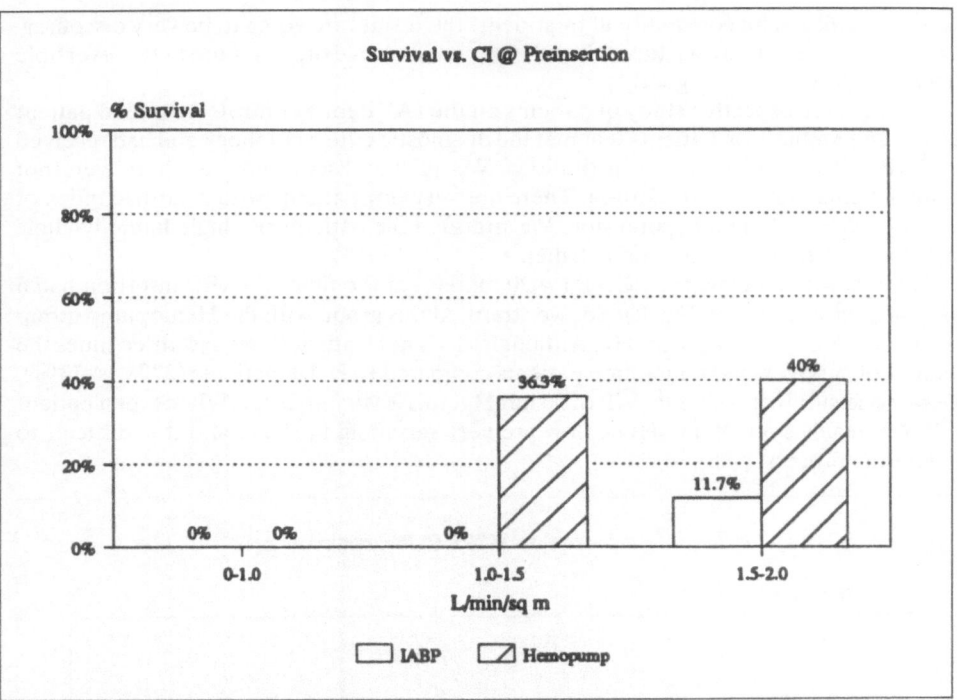

Fig. 3. Relationship between survival of patients treated with IABP or Hemopump and pre-insertion cardiac index (CI expressed in L/min/sq m).

There are two equations for the work indexes: one is to look at the work in a given stroke (left-ventricular stroke work index (LVSWI); the second is to look at ventricular power (left-ventricular work index (LVWI) which is work per unit time. We chose the convention of power. The total left-venticular power happens to be the difference in work per minute between the aorta and the ventricle and is expressed as PCWP + MAP × CI × 13.6 = LVWI.

A normal LVWI is about 3500 gmm/m²/min. A significant degree of shock is present when the LVWI is < 2000 gmm/m²/min. Hemopump patients had to have a work index of < 1500 gmm/m²/min to be candidates, based on their pre-admission criteria. LVWI is the most discriminate indicator of the degrees of shock. It is possible to have a CI that is very good, or a PCWP that is very good, and still have a very bad LVWI. The LVWI is a very good global predictor of how sick someone is and how likely they are to survive. When looking at patients with a LVWI of less than 1500 gmm/m²/min., the Hemopump survival was 40% versus the IABP survival which was about 7%, chi square analysis revealed $p < .0001$.

Figure 4 shows survival resp. Hemopump vs. IABP as a function of LVWI; 0–500, 500–1000, and 1000–1500. We had better survival in all groups compared to the retrospective IABP patients. The second point is that Hemopump patients did better if their work indexes were higher when they began assistance. If one waits for a patient to get below 1000 before deciding to use the Hemopump, survival falls significantly. If the patients had a work index of over 1000, they had a very respectable chance of a 30-day survival (60%).

44

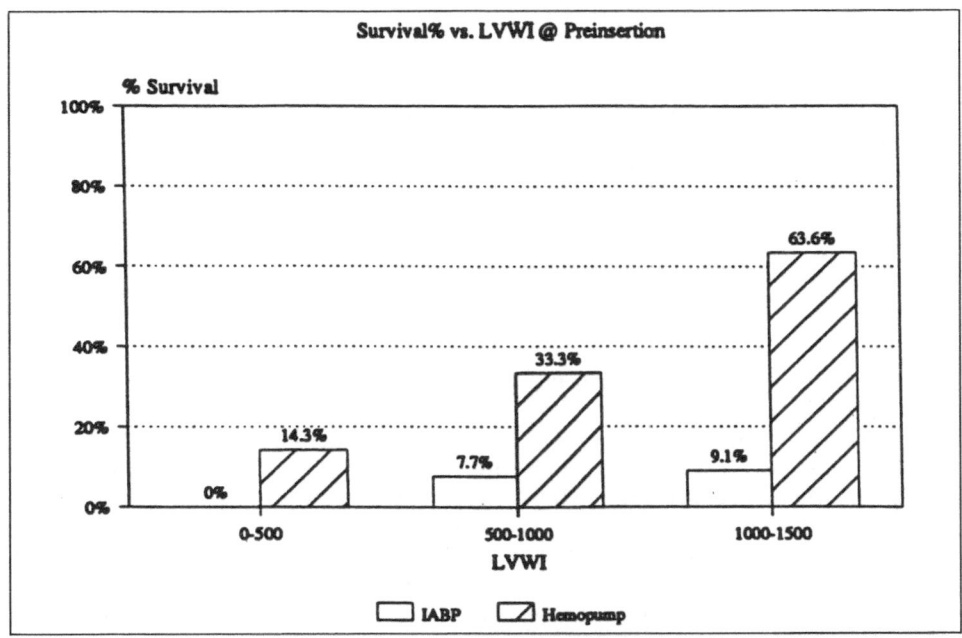

Fig. 4 Relationship between survival of patients treated with IABP or Hemopump and pre-insertion left ventricular work index (LVWI expressed in gmm/m²/ min).

Figure 5 shows the distribution of patients after 24 h. If the CI was < 2 or the PCWP was > 20, the chance for survival was very poor. So, if you cannot get the CI > 2 and the PCWP < 20 within 24 h, the patient is likely not recoverable or the device is not doing what it is supposed to do.

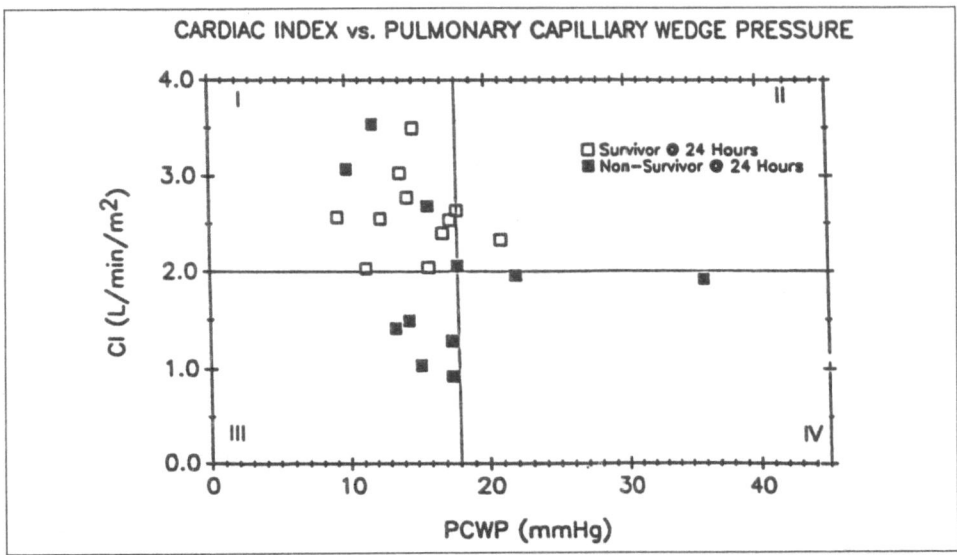

Fig. 5 Outcome of patients after 24 h of treatment with IABP or Hemopump in relation to cardiac index (CI) and pulmonary wedge pressure (PCWP).

Hints

In closing, we would like to focus on some important hints:
- Due to the fact that you may only do 10 Hemopump cases per year, continuing educational classes must be set up in order to keep personnel trained.
- Right to Left shunting will be recognized by watching the venous saturation via an oximetric catheter or by doing spot checks of venous samples.
- Dr. Frazier advocates a "sparing use of heparin". We are not willing to entirely agree with that. We believe it is appropriate to run patients with ACT's at 1.5–2 times control and *very* important to have them anticoagulated during the insertion. That includes the time advancing it up and over the aortic arch and to the beginning of pumping. You cannot have static blood on a foreign surface, no matter how anticoagulated, and expect to avoid thrombus formation! So, continue with heparin flushes during inserton.
- Dr. Richard Smalling (Univ. of Texas) is doing something different from other investigators. He has had successful insertion in 13 out of 13 cases. He uses a peripheral angioplasty balloon (10–12 mm) to blindly predilate the femoral and iliac system before he tries to place the Hemopump. He puts in a standard guidewire through an introducer sheath, then passes up a large (10–12 mm) balloon. He inflates the balloon and pulls back until he encounters resistance. He assumes the resistance occurs when the balloon is at the bifurcation of the aorta and then serially dilates the balloon slowly coming out of the iliac system. He must be doing something right; it seems to work – even in small people.

Investigational trials of the Hemopump at the Texas Heart Institute: practical issues

O. H. Frazier

Texas Heart Institute, Houston, Texas, USA

Introduction

When we were first introduced to the Hemopump, we were skeptical about it. We feared that the device would cause hemolysis, as well as other problems. In fact, we told Dr. Wampler that we did not think it would work, but we did the initial animal experiments anyway. To paraphrase the famous Frenchman Claude Bernard, however, "You have to decide on the experiment and hang your ideas outside the laboratory, do the experiment, and see what nature says, not what you think." We did the animal experiments, and they went very well, as has been reported in the literature (5). We saw no abnormality in plasma-free hemoglobin levels or hematologic profiles (Figs. 1, 2). The animals tolerated the intraventricular device very well.

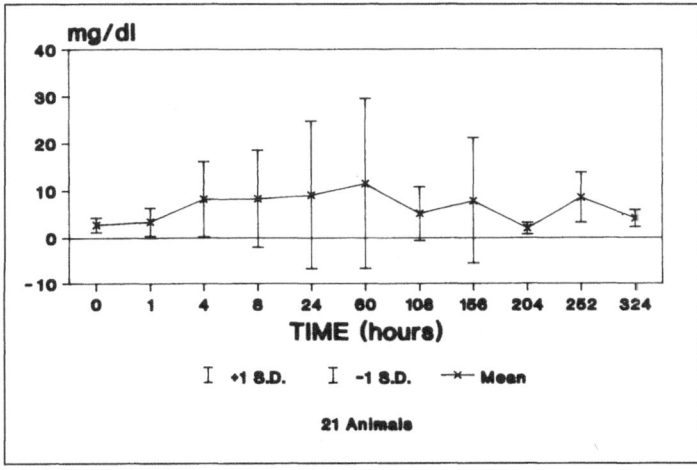

Fig. 1. The average plasma free hemoglobin levels for 21 animals (from (5)).

Other investigators voiced concerns about blood being sucked from the coronary arteries. The Hemopump provides intraventricular ejection, the coronary arteries fill normally and the aortic valve is not injured.

Design and operation

In comparison with other left-ventricular assist devices that require direct cardiac cannulation, the Hemopump is much easier to use (1). It can be inserted by advancing the cannula assembly through a graft sewn to the femoral artery, as was done to insert the

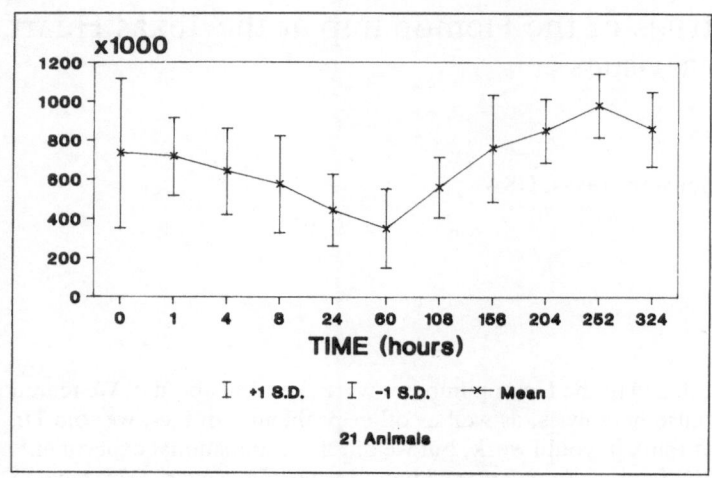

Fig. 2. Platelet history of 21 implant animals (from (1)).

early nonpulsatile intraortic balloon pump before the percutaneous device was available. The Hemopump cable that exits the groin is actually much smaller than the diameter of the balloon pump.

To properly place the device, the silicone inflow cannula is advanced across the aortic valve, so that its tip rests within the left ventricle, and the impeller lies just distal to the subclavian artery. Placement must be verified by use of fluoroscopy.

After Hemopump support is instituted and the heart begins to recover function, the heart may eject the pump or the cable may bend, resulting in breakage. To avoid complications like these, the cable must be secured by tying umbilical tape firmly around the silastic guards. Once the pump is in place and working, it is safe, and few problems occur.

The ascending aortic approach has been used to insert the Hemopump (1). A shorter cannula is needed for this approach, but in early cases, cable breakages occurred. With further design modification, we hope to resume using the aortic approach, which would make using the Hemopump feasible intraoperatively. The retroperitoneal approach by way of the distal abdominal aorta is better for small patients or for patients with peripheral vascular disease, when difficulty passing the device is anticipated.

Current clinical applications

Through animal and clinical studies, we have found that many of our fears about the Hemopump were unfounded. Patients have not experienced thromboembolic complications or excessive hemolysis. Patients who have increased plasma-free hemoglobin levels during support are the ones who have been on prolonged cardiopulmonary bypass, a known cause of hemolysis.

Patients who do not require cardiopulmonary bypass before Hemopump insertion have relatively normal plasma-free hemoglobin levels. Finally, we have also found that the Hemopump does not affect coronary circulation, and no problems related to placing the pump/cannula assembly across the aortic valve have occurred in patients or in animals.

Our experience with the Hemopump shows that it is a good therapeutic option when the potential for heart recovery exists. In general, patients who are placed on the device have improvement in cardiac index, left-ventricular work index, and arterial pressure, as well as a reduction in capillary wedge pressure. Many patients have remained awake and alert during support.

We would now like to describe cases representative of the various indications for Hemopump support.

The first case involved a man who had undergone heart transplantation. We had reduced his immunosuppression when pneumonia developed. Within several days of operation, he suffered severe rejection, and he was placed on OKT3. Despite medical therapy, the patients's condition continued to deteriorate, so we wanted to support him with the Hemopump. After we explained to the family what we were doing and what our hopes were, we inserted the device. By the time the patient had been transferred to the recovery room, his circulation was being well maintained by the pump. No pulsatile flow occurred for 6 to 8 h. When cardiac ejection resumed, we were trying to assess when to remove the Hemopump. Nature made the decision for us – the cable broke and we were forced to remove it. It must be mentioned that we were using an early version of the device that had problems when even slight angulations occurred. This problem has been addressed and is no longer an issue, but minimizing angulation is necessary, since the device operates at 25,000 revolutions per minute. This patient is a long-term survivor.

The second patient we would like to describe was a man who had had an acute myocardial infarction. His cardiac output was very low, so we inserted the Hemopump. He had excellent hemodynamic recovery during 4 days of support. Unfortunately, the patient had global cardiac dysfunction, and his wife refused the option of transplantation because he had been ill a long time. The device was removed, and the patient died 2 h later.

Another patient we treated with the Hemopump was a 71-year-old woman who went into severe cardiogenic shock during a procedure in the catheterization laboratory. She underwent emergency coronary artery bypass surgery and could not be weaned from cardiopulmonary bypass. The Hemopump supported this patient 2 days, after which she was successfully weaned. She is still alive, which certainly would not have happened without the Hemopump.

As we have stated, the Hemopump is designed for use in the potentially recoverable heart. Thus, the ideal patient population includes heart transplant recipients. The Hemopump can be used to provide circulatory support when severe allograft rejection occurs or when a donor heart fails to function immediately after transplant. In each of these cases where we have instituted Hemopump support, the heart has recovered. The Hemopump is much less invasive than other left ventricular assist devices and, because it is inserted by way of the femoral artery, it does not necessitate cannulating the heart of the immunosuppressed patient.

The future

The Hemopump has proved safe, with minimal or no risk, when used properly in well-selected patients. The U.S. Food and Drug Administration has currently set restrictions for the Hemopump during the approval process and limits the durations of support to 7 days. However, we continue to evaluate further indications for its use.

Our experience shows that high-risk surgical patients may benefit from being placed directly on Hemopump support, altogether bypassing support with the intraaortic balloon pump. At the Texas Heart Institute in 1988, 175 patients were placed on balloon pump support. Of these patients, 20 died because they could not be weaned from cardiopulmonary bypass. An additional 24 patients died of severe hepatic and renal insufficiency within 24 h of operation. Whereas the intraaortic balloon pump augments existing heart function, the Hemopump can provide adequate end-organ perfusion.

For carefully selected cardiac transplant patients, the Hemopump may prove satisfactory in staged transplant procedures (2). This possibility may materialize in Europe, where no restrictions have been placed on duration of support and the waiting period for a donor heart is much shorter than that in the U.S.A.

Finally, the Hemopump may be used for cardiopulmonary bypass. We recently treated a young man who suffered dissection of the left anterior descending artery during a procedure in the catheterization laboratory. The Hemopump was inserted immediately, after which the patient was taken to the operating room for coronary artery bypass. The operation was accomplished with no other means of circulatory support but the Hemopump, with the flow rate at 3.5 L/min. This decompressed the left ventricle, and the operation was completed without a great deal of difficulty. Hemopump support was continued for 3 days after the operation, with the patient gradually being weaned from support as his own cardiac function recovered. He had an uneventful recovery and returned home 2.5 weeks later.

Conclusion

The Hemopump, capable of providing flows of 3.0 to 3.5 l, can be used with little risk in selected patients (3, 4). Furthermore, it is easier to implant than other left-ventricular assist devices. The Hemopump is more akin to the intraaortic balloon pump. No thoracic incisions are necessary to insert the Hemopump. It can decompress the left ventricle and works well as long as the cable is not kinked. Finally, the Hemopump can support approximately 80% of the normal function of the adult heart and will allow for survival and left ventricular recovery, if recovery is possible. The Hemopump is intended for use only when the hope of myocardial salvage exists. In addition, there is a limitation of inserting the pump through the femoral artery in patients with small vessels or with atherosclerotic occlusive disease because of the size of the cannula (21 F). In these patients, the abdominal aorta has been used as an alternative approach.

References

1. Duncan JM, Frazier OH, Radovancevic B, Velebit V (1989) Implantation techniques for the Hemopump. Ann Thorac Surg 48: 733–735
2. Frazier OH, Macris MP, Wampler RK, Duncan JM, Sweeney MS, Fuqua JM (1990) Treatment of cardiac allograft failure by use on an intraaortic axial flow pump. J Heart Transplant 9: 408–414
3. Frazier OH, Radovancevic B (1990) Ventricular assist devices. Cardiac Surgery: State of the Art Reviews 4: 335–347
4. Frazier OH, Wampler RK, Duncan JM, et al (1990) First human use of the Hemopump, a catheter-mounted ventricular assist device. Ann Thorac Surg 49: 299–304
5. Wampler RK, Moise JC, Frazier OH, Olsen DB (1988) In vivo evaluation of a peripheral vascular access axial flow blood pump. ASAIO Transactions 34: 450–454

Succes and failure of the Hemopump: a critical analysis

U. Mees, P. Sergeant, W. Daenen and W. Flameng

University Clinic Gasthuisberg, Department of Cardiac Surgery, Leuven, Belgium

Introduction

As with all new circulatory assist devices, we have to search for the optimal indications, the limitations of the system, and the possible complications. Therefore we have to deal with a certain learning process in order to finally obtain stable results.

Up to now, the group of patients supported with the Hemopump is rather small and, therefore, it is impossible to give a general survey of correct indications, limitations, and peculiarities of the system and of their real incidences. By supporting a patient with the hemopump, there are a few typical and specific tricks and pitfalls which one has to be aware of. For that reason, we will try to demonstrate, by means of two cases, a few of these problems and discuss them.

Clinical material

Case 1

History: A 56-year-old man with a history of an acute myocardial infarction in 1969 underwent, in 1975, coronary artery bypass grafting combined with left-ventricular aneurysmectomy. He developed, 14 years after surgery, another unstable angina syndrome.

The night before the re-operation was scheduled, he again suffered from prolonged chest pain with significant ECG changes and his complaints were refractory to augmentation of the classical pharmacological treatment (calcium antagonists, intravenous nitro-glycerine-infusion, β-blocking agents, and heparinization).

Hemodynamically, the patient deteriorated very quickly and when he arrived in the operating theater he was in severe cardiogenic shock and needed cardiopulmonary resuscitation. Because severe adhesions of the heart and great vessels, resulting from the previous operation, could be expected, and because of the external cardiac massage, we connected the cardiopulmonary bypass via the femoral artery and vein before performing the sternotomy.

Coronary bypass surgery was succesfully carried out and revascularization was complete. However, the patient could not be weaned from cardiopulmonary bypass because of low cardiac output. The first attempt was made under maximal inotropic support but after a few minutes a severe low cardiac output state developed and we decided to reperfuse the patient on cardiopulmonary bypass. After more than 1 h of reperfusion, we made another attempt to wean the patient. This time we noticed a somewhat improved pumpfunction, but we still needed maximal inotropic support and atrio-ventricular sequential pacing. Ten minutes later, again signs of left-ventricular failure appeared:

cardiac index < 2.0 l/min/m² with a left atrial pressure > 20 mm Hg. Again we placed the patient on full cardiopulmonary bypass and we decided, after a total pump run of nearly 5 h, to insert the Hemopump by means of fluoroscopy via the contralateral femoral artery, and to try to wean the patient during Hemopump support.

Recovery of hemodynamics: Within a few minutes after the Hemopump was started, we could succesfully wean the patient from the CPB. However, the left ventricle was clearly pump-dependent. We measured a total cardiac output of 4.5 l/min, with a calculated flow through the Hemopump (when it was on full speed) of 3.5 l/min. So the left ventricle of the patient only provided an output of 1 l/min. In contrast, the right ventricle was doing well. This could be evaluated devisu and also by trans-esophageal echocardiography.

During the postoperative phase, we observed a continuous improvement of the hemodynamic status of the patient. Total cardiac output increased from 4.2 l/min to

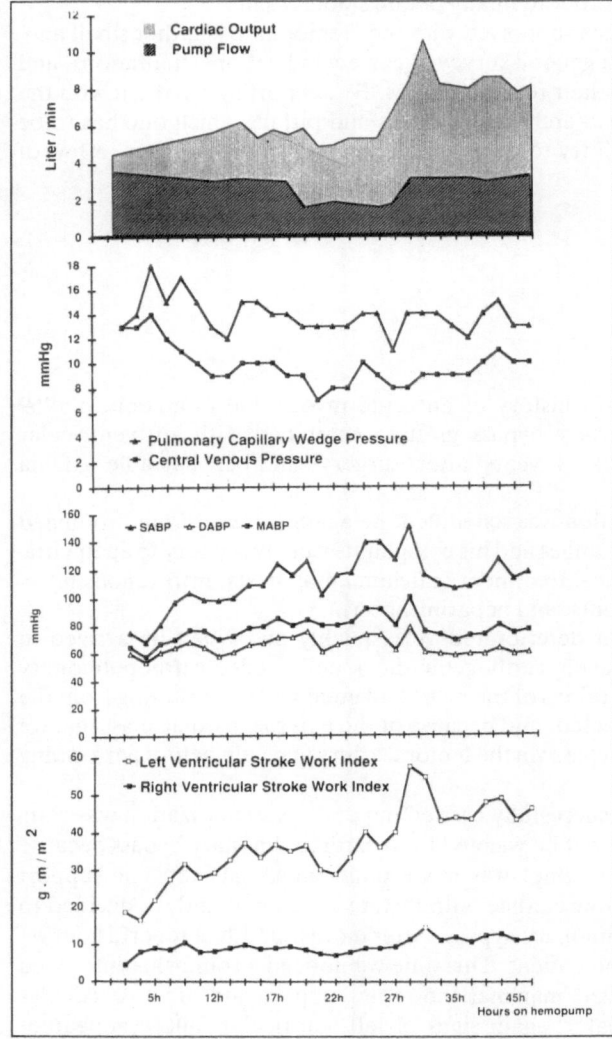

Fig. 1. Hemodynamic performance. Cardiac output, pulmonary capillary wedge pressure, differential pressure, and left-ventricular stroke work index, during Hemopump support.

8.0 l/min with a contstant contribution of the Hemopump (see Fig. 1). A decompression of the left ventricle was noticed, which is expressed as a drop of the pulmonary capillary wedge pressure: from18 mmHg to12 mmHg (see Fig. 1). Also, the central venous pressure was declining.

There was a restoration of the differential pressure between systolic and diastolic arterial blood pressure when the patient was on Hemopump support (see Fig. 1), which was also expressed by an increase in left ventricle stroke work index during the Hemopump run (see Fig. 1).

As the left-ventricular output improved, also metabolic recovery was noticed and the patient was weaned from the Hemopump after 52 h of support. This weaning process was performed gradually.

By measuring total cardiac output with the thermodilution method, and by substracting the calculated pump output, we have an idea of the output of the left ventricle itself. As the left-ventricular output improved, the Hemopump speed was reduced step by step, and this over a period of several hours. By doing so, a greater and greater fraction of total left-ventricular output was produced by the left-ventricular muscle itself (see Fig. 2).

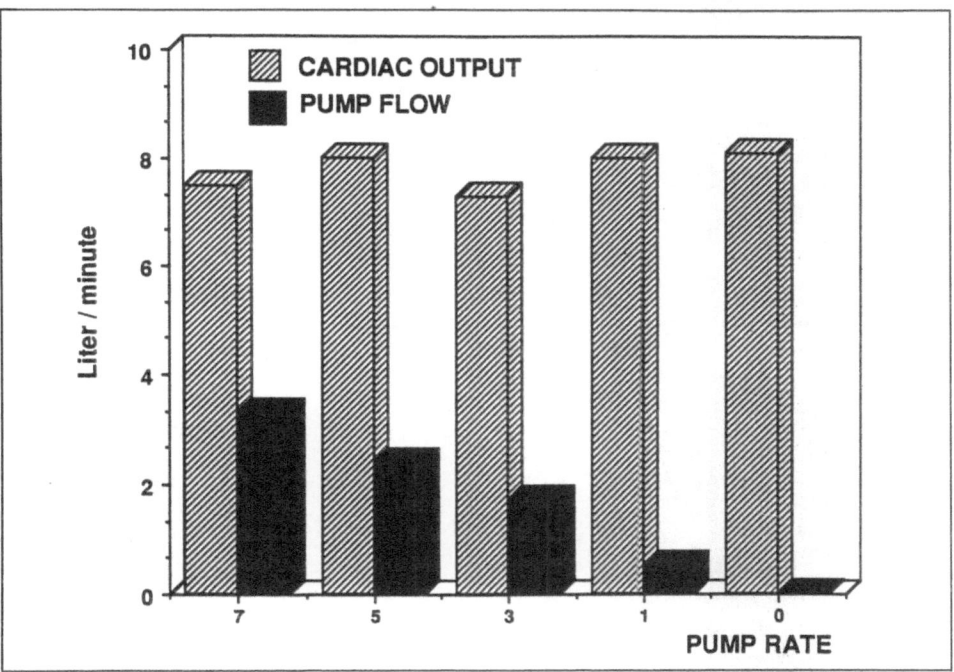

Fig. 2. Hemodynamic performance during weaning from the Hemopump support system.

During the weaning phase cardiac output remained stable and only a little increase was observed in pulmonary capillary wedge pressure. Thus, the patient was succesfully weaned.

Metabolic recovery: During the time the patient was on Hemopump support and during the postpump period, there was not only a significant improvement of cardiac function, but also of renal and liver function. Both organ systems are very sensitive to a period of shock.

– *Renal function:* During Hemopump support there was a decrease in the creatinine level (from 1.6 mg% to 1.2 mg%) and a slight but not significant rise in blood urea nitrogen (from 25 mg% to 40 mg%) which remained still in the normal range. In the post-pump phase there was an initial rise in the absolute values of both parameters but after a few days they reached again preoperative levels (see figure 3).

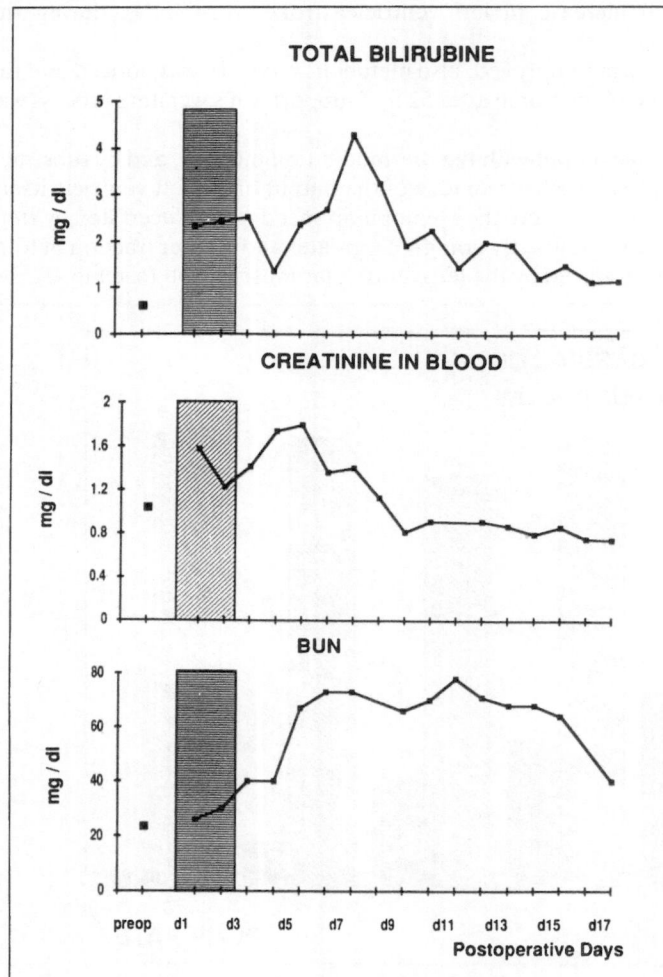

Fig. 3. Preservation of the renal function (creatinine in blood and blood urea nitrogen) and liver function (total bilirubine level in blood) during Hemopump support and in the post-pump period: creatinine in blood (shaded part = period on Hemopump support).

– *Liver function:* In this case the Hemopump was also able to preserve liver function after a period of severe cardiogenic shock and prolonged cardiopulmonary bypass.

Initially, the total bilirubine levels were elevated (up to 4.5 mg%) as compared to the preoperative value, but after a few days they again reached normal preoperative levels (see Figure 3).

Hemostasis: During Hemopump support fibrinogen levels dropped to less than 2 g/l, but in the postpump period fibrinogen levels were restored to normal (between 4 and 6 g/l).

54

Our anticoagulation management of a patient on Hemopump support is as follows. In case of postcardiotomy cardiogenic shock patients are of course fully heparinized for the cardiopulmonary bypass period. Heparin is completely antagonized by the administration of protamine, coagulation factors and platelets to become a normal coagulation state. Therefore, administration of heparin is stopped for several hours (up to 12 h maximally). When the patient shows normal thrombus formation the administration of heparin is started again under guidance of the activated clotting time untill it reaches two times the normal value.

Blood elements: Only minimal trauma to blood elements was noticed.

Due to prolonged cardiopulmonary bypass there was a drop in hemoglobin (8.5 gr/dl) as compared to the preoperative value (14.4 gr/dl). Blood was transfused to maintain an acceptable level of hemoglobin (see Fig. 4). Values of free hemoglobin were elevated (34 mg%) due to a prolonged cardiopulmonary bypass. The free hemoglobin level dropped to normal values (2 mg%) after the cardiopulmonary bypass was stopped and while the patient was on Hemopump support.

A drop in platelets was seen during Hemopump support (50000/ml) and the first 5 postpump days despite a significant amount of thrombocyte transfusions (see Fig. 4).

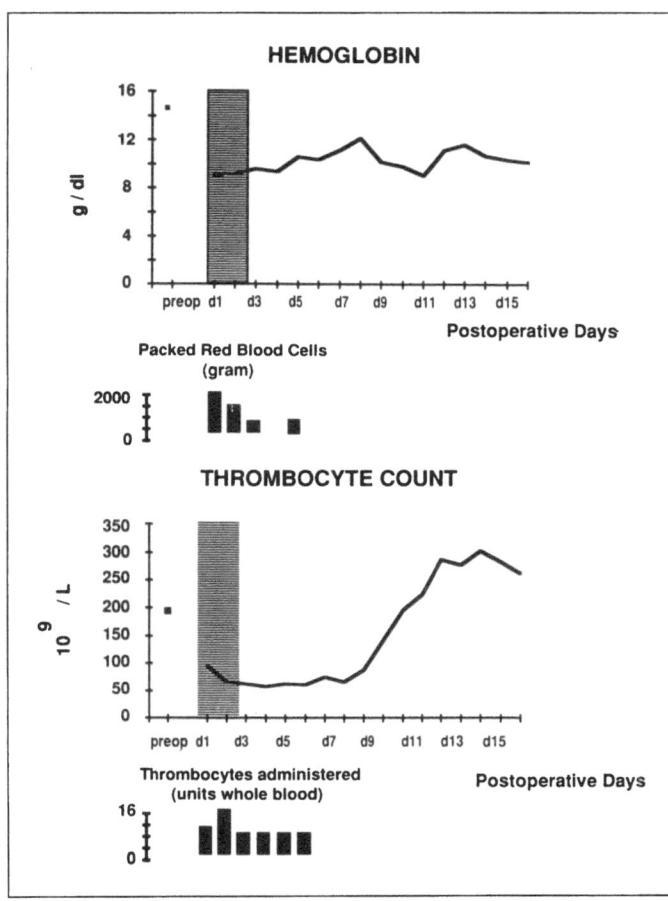

Fig. 4. Upper panel: Hemoglobin level during Hemopump support and in the postpump period. In the lower part of the figure: the amount of administered red blood cells.
Lower panel: Thrombocytes count during Hemopump support and in the postpump period. In the lower part of the figure: the amount of administered thrombocytes (shaded part = period on Hemopump support).

55

Clinical outcome: This patient recovered and was discharged from the hospital 15 days after removal of the Hemopump.

Case 2

History: A-68-year old woman had a history of acute inferoposterior myocardial infarction with mitral insufficiency due to rupture of a papillary muscle. During the following days she developed a hemodynamic deterioration with signs of left-ventricular failure. Five days after the onset of the infarction the patient was transferred to our service for mitral valve replacement and coronary artery bypass grafting.

When the patient arrived in our institution she was in a low cardiac output state and underwent emergency surgery.

After bypass grafting to the left anterior descending and the posterior descending coronary artery, combined with a mitral valve replacement (Björk Shiley valve No. 25), weaning from cardiopulmonary bypass was difficult and required maximal inotropic drug therapy. The hemodynamic response however was minimal and associated with a severe compromized cardiac function (cardiac index < 1.8 l/min/m^2), pulmonary edema, and hypotension.

The Hemopump system was inserted through the femoral artery.

The placement of the Hemopump was controlled with trans-esophageal echocardiography. Immediately after starting Hemopump support, there was an improvement of the hemodynamic status of the patient. Cardiac output went up from 2.0 l/min to 4.8 l/min and there was a drop in the left filling pressures: from 25 mmHg to 14 mmHg.

Postoperative problems: Two hours after placing the Hemopump there was a sudden loss of current pulsatility on the console. A transoesophagal echography showed that the cannula was spontaneuosly expelled from the left ventricle, which was confirmed by an x-Ray of the chest.

It was possible to replace the cannula in the LV which was performed under echographic control. This turned out to be difficult. Obviously, the flexible beveled tip of the cannula was kinked, there was a bend in the cannula and the pump screw itself was situated in the aortic arch and not in the transition area between the aortic arch and the descending aorta. The bend radius of the flexible drive shaft was too short, which significantly increased the stress in the flexible shaft and resulted in a shortened shaft life. After 21 h of Hemopump support a fracture of the drive cable occurred. An x-Ray of the chest (see Fig. 5) revealed the malpositioning of the cannula which resulted hemodynamically in a drop in cardiac output and arterial pressure and in elevation of the filling pressures (see Fig. 6).

The pump needed to be replaced.

During replacement of the pump, there was migration of thrombus material from the graft into the distal part of the femoral artery which resulted in severe limb ischemia. It was decided to remove the Hemopump to allow performance of a thrombectomy on the ischemic limb. Meanwhile, pharmacological support was started using high doses of positive inotropic drugs. Initially, this was efficient so that another replacement of the Hemopump could be postponed.

Clinical outcome: With the use of positive inotropic support the patient did well hemodynamically, but developed sepsis. Unfortunately, two days after removal of the Hemopump the patient died in septic shock.

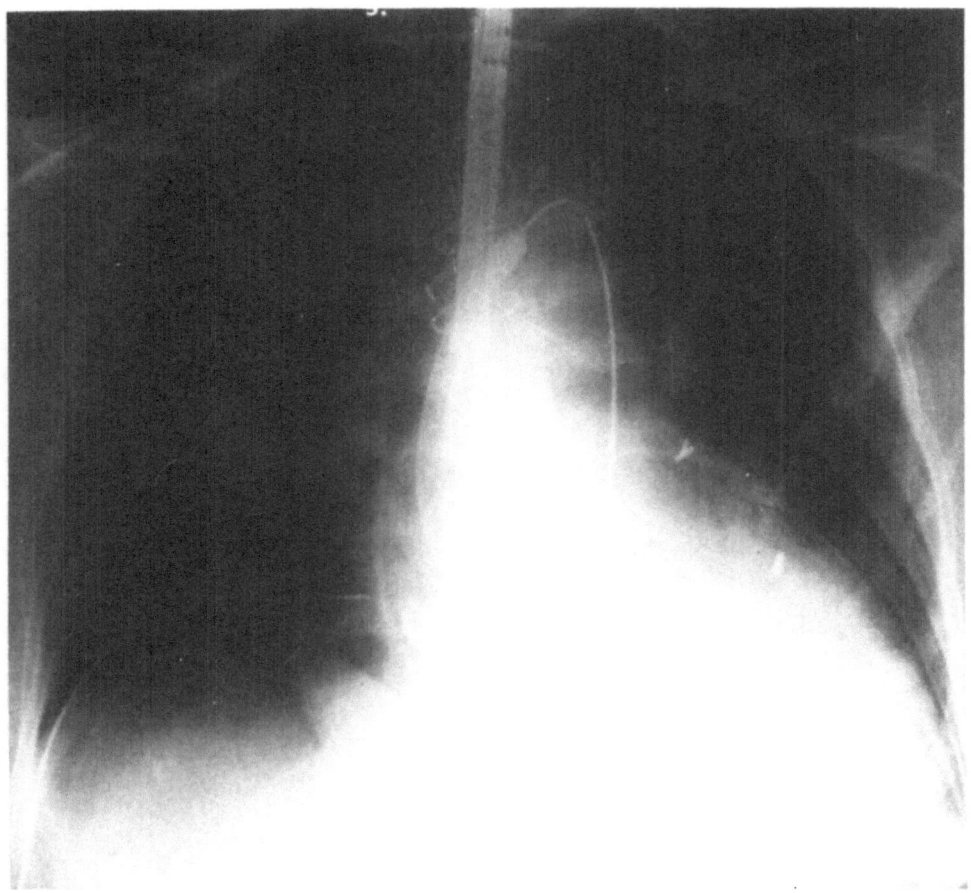

Fig. 5. Chest x-ray indicating fracture of the cable of the Hemopump.

Discussion

As with all the patients in the postcardiotomy cardiogenic shock group we have to deal with the main question of whether or not the myocardium is reversibly or irreversibly damaged.

The differentiation between reversible, transient postischemic dysfunction of the myocardium (often referred to as "stunning") and necrosis is difficult in the early stages and clinically useful parameters are not yet available. Indirect evidence like the absence of preoperative signs of previous myocardial necrosis, the absence of significant washout of cardiac enzymes, etc., can suggest reversibility. The decision to accept a patient as a candidate for left-ventricular assist, however, will always remain based on subjective parameters.

In the first case, we certainly were dealing with myocardial stunning, because by unloading the left ventricle and consequently diminishing myocardial oxygen consumption and work, time for functional recovery of the hypokinetic myocardium was provided.

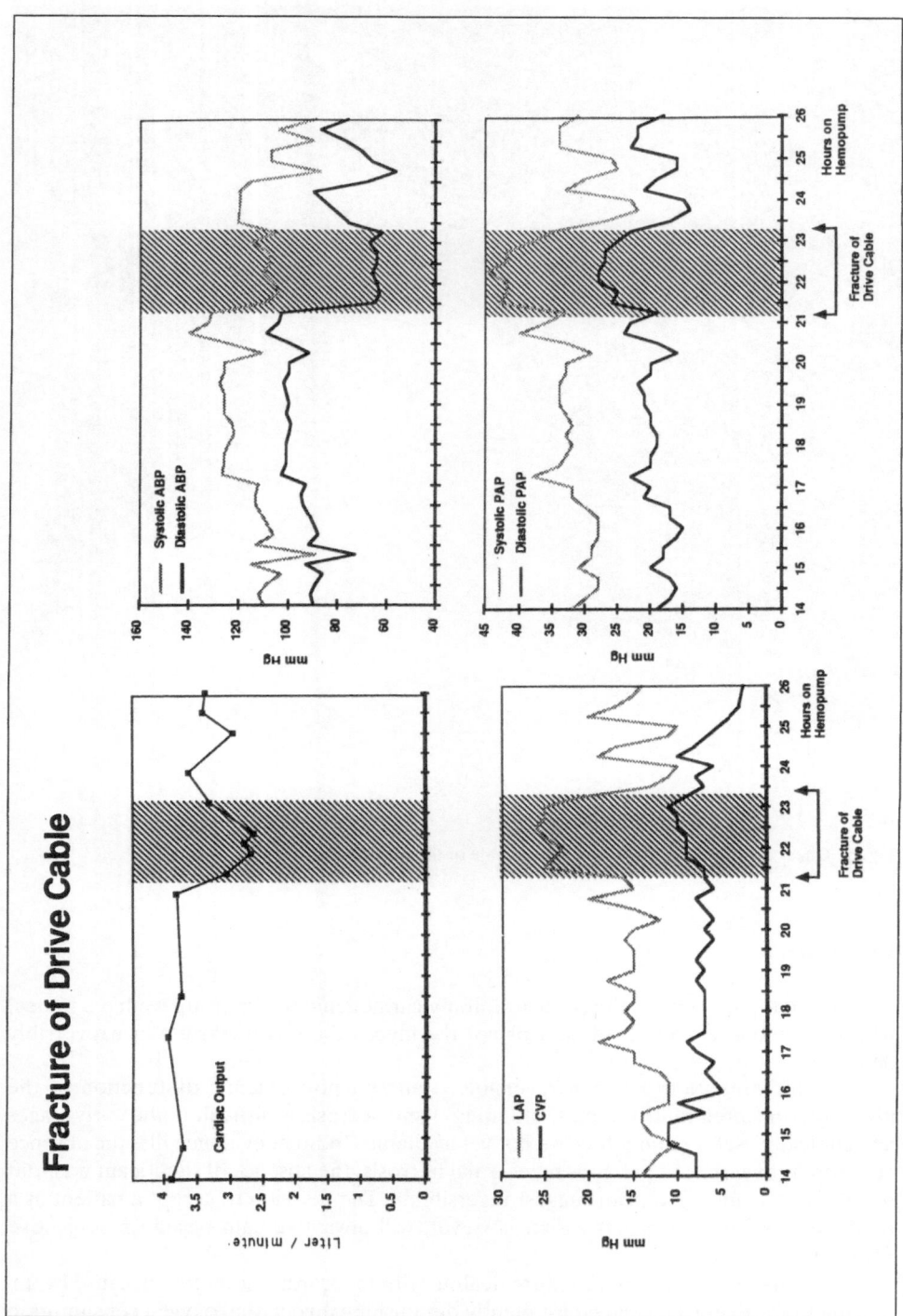

Fig. 6 Hemodynamic performance during Hemopump support: fracture of the drive cable.

From the hemodynamic point of view, we can conclude that this co-axial pump system is effective in supporting the transiently failing myocardium and in adequately perfusing the vital organs. Therefore it may be a lifesaving support system.

On the other hand, a lot of practical problems may be related to the lack of experience with the use of this co-axial pump system or to inadequate monitoring of the functions of the device, which was illustrated by the second case.

Pitfalls due to *inexperience* may be an expulsion of the cannula and fracture of the drive cable which could be avoided by exact placement of the cannula. In our opinion, it is not possible to do so with the use of echocardiography alone; fluoroscopy is definitivly needed.

Ischemia of the leg was only seen after exchange of the cannula, and is most probably due to peripheral embolization of thrombotic material originating from the femoral prosthetic graft which often contains a thrombus.

Inadequate monitoring possibilities of the pump system

Instantaneous flows in the cannula are not indicated in the Hemopump system as it is actually used. The output of pump flow on the console for a certain mean arterial pressure is a calculated flow, but not an actual flow. In fact, it is perfectly possible to read a certain flow rate on the console while the cannula is completely obstructed by a thrombus.

Nevertheless, this type of co-axial support system is a promising device which has the potential of a moderate assist system. However, further clinical experience is needed for an overall judgement.

References

1. Duncan JM, Frazier OH, Radorvancevic B, Velebit N (1989) Implantation techniques for the Hemopump. Ann Thorac Surg 48: 733–5
2. Pae WE (1987) Current indications and results. Trans am soc artif intern organs XXXIII: 3–7
3. Pae WE, Pierce WS, Pennock JL, Campbell DB, Waldhausen JA (1987) Long term results of ventricular assist pumping in postcardiotomy cardiogenic shock. J Thorac Cardiovasc Surg 93: 434–41
4. Pennington DG, Copeland JG (1989) Circulatory support 1988. Topical meeting of the society of thoracic surgeons. Ann Thorac Surg 47: 73–178
5. Unger F (1989) Assisted Circulation 3. Springer, New York Berlin Heidelberg, pp 621

Clinical results of Hemopump support in surgical cases

O. Jegaden

Hôpital Vasculaire Louis Pradel, Lyon, France

Introduction

The principle of the Hemopump is to provide a temporary circulatory support in patients with acute cardiac failure. The Hemopump works by unloading the left ventricle and, therefore, by protecting the myocardium. Its mean output ranging from 2 to 4 l/min assures a satisfactory cerebral and visceral perfusion, as demonstrated in the experimental set-up (see chapter 4). In addition, the ability to implant the device without invasion of the mediastinum and surgical trauma to the heart may decrease the incidence of infection and increase the possibility of myocardial recuperation.

Generally, indications of the Hemopump are emergency situations, therefore, the surgical procedure for insertion of the device must be easy, fast, and safe: We developed the femoral insertion without graft, with guidance of the canula by a vascular guide and catheter, allowing easy placement of the tip in the left ventricle.

According to our initial experience with the Hemopump, this device provides effective left-ventricular assistance. However, some limitations of the system will determine the indications of this type of circulatory support.

Hemopump insertion technique

The most common method of Hemopump implantation is by the left femoral artery approach. Under anesthesia, the common femoral artery is exposed and then clamped. After arteriotomy, a guide wire and a 5F catheter are passed through the distal hole of the

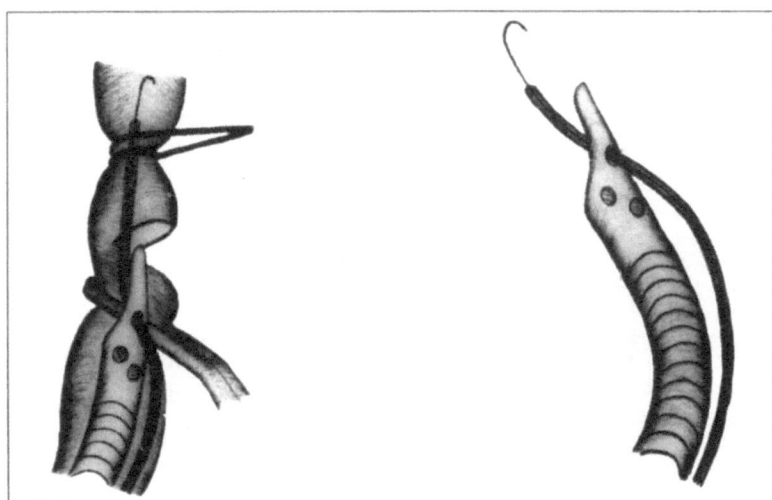

Fig. 1.

canula and introduced into the femoral artery up to the aorta (Fig. 1). Then the canula is introduced into the femoral artery and is pushed into the aorta, guided by the vascular catheter (Fig. 2). Retrograde bleeding through the canula and pumphead is avoided by a silicone occluder of the outflow port of the canula. The occluder is removed just before the drive cable is inserted into the vessel lumen. The femoral artery is then clamped with a silicone loop around the artery, and it is possible to move the Hemopump inserted with the drive cable without bleeding.

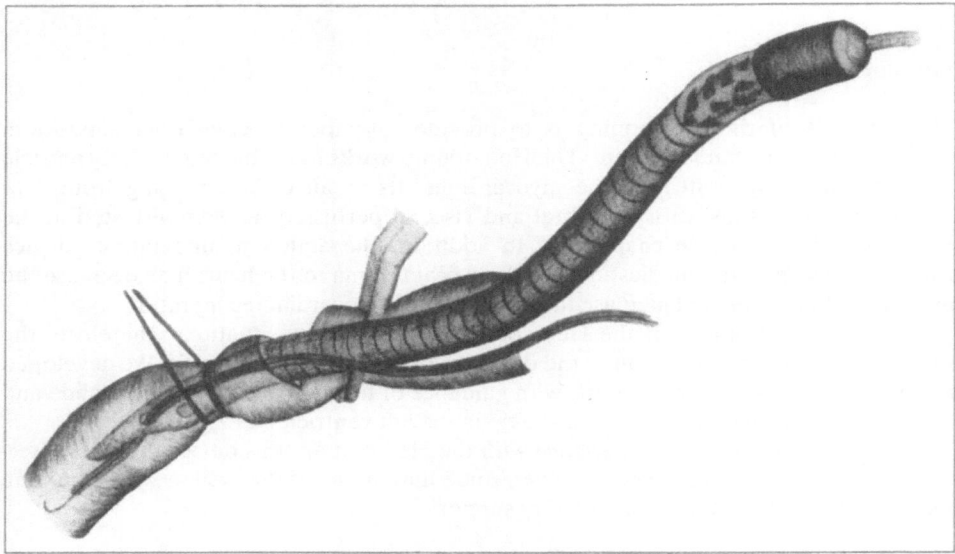

Fig. 2.

Under fluoroscopic guidance, the vascular guide is pushed up to the left ventricle, then the catheter is pushed on the guide, then the canula of the Hemopump is pushed on the catheter up to the left ventricle (Fig. 3). This guidance technique is very effective for the progression of the canula into the aorta, without false route or arterial traumatism, especially when the arteries are of marginal size. The passing through the aortic valve and

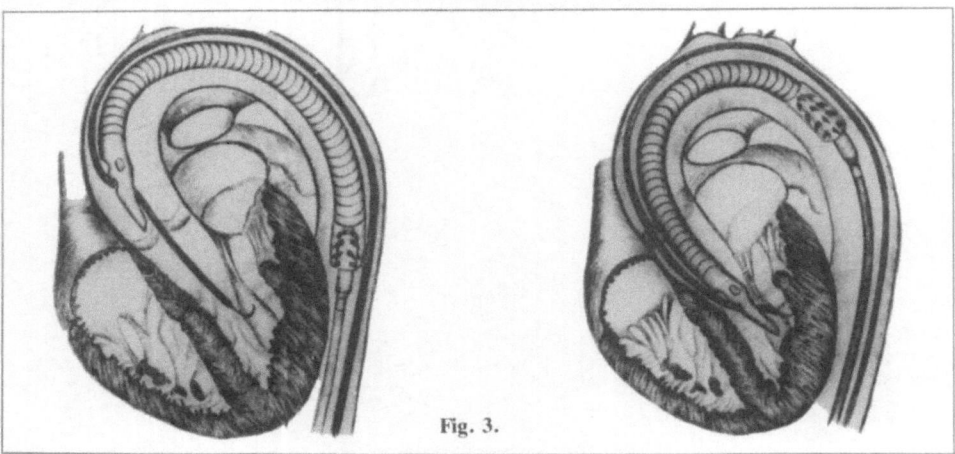

Fig. 3.

the good positioning of the canula into the left ventricle are easier to perform; the ejection of the canula out of the left ventricle is also prevented by this technique. When the position of the canula in the left ventricle is satisfactory, first the catheter is removed and then the guide.

The pump is activated as soon as the tip of the canula is in the ascending aorta. A few separate sutures are performed to close the femoral arteriotomy around the drive cable. The silicone plug fixed around the drive cable close to the artery is attached to the tissue to prevent bleeding or canula moving.

This Hemopump insertion technique is easy, safe, and fast to use in all cases, especially when fluoroscopic guidance can be avoided in a patient who has undergone sternotomy. In all other cases, fluoroscopic guidance is useful. In one case we used an echographic guidance with good result. In our opinion, this may be a good alternative.

Anticoagulative therapy

Heparin is administered intravenously to maintain an activated clotting time of 1.5 to 2 times control. If the patient had postoperative blood loss or coagulopathy, anticoagulative therapy is omitted until hemostasis is achieved.

Hemodynamic monitoring and management

All patients are monitored with continuous electrocardiographic measurements, radial arterial lines, and a pulmonary artery catheter. Cardiac output determinations are made using the standard thermodilution techniques. All attempts are made to provide optimal pump flow, including maintainance of adequate intravascular volume and left-ventricular filling pressure, and by reducing systemic vascular resistance. Additionally, the use of inotropic agents is minimized.

Hematologic studies

All patients are carefully monitored for rheologic abnormalities. Peripheral blood smears are also routinely examined for evidence of hemolysis.

Device weaning and removal

Once the patient's heart has adequately recovered, pump speed is gradually reduced from 7 to 1. The pump is not stopped until shortly before removal. Heparin is not reversed. After removal of the device, the cannulation site is inspected for evidence of endotheleal damage or thrombus formation. The arteriotomy is then repaired using separate sutures.

Clinical experience

Five patients in cardiogenic shock were treated with the Hemopump. These patient had acute myocardial infarction (n = 3), failure to wean from CPB (n = 1), and cardiac allograft rejection (n = 1). Failure of femoral insertion occurred in two other patients who had diffuse arteriosclerotic desease; the indications for the use of the Hemopump was failure to wean from cardiopulmonary bypass.

Acute myocardial infarction

Case 1: A 64-year-old man had severe three-vessel disease. His left-ventricular ejection fraction was 66%. Percutaneous transluminal angioplasty of the left anterior descending coronary artery was attempted. Unfortunately, the procedure was complicated by left main dissection, and cardiac arrest occurred. The patient was resuscitated and a Hemopump was placed through the left femoral approach in the catheterization laboratory. As soon as the Hemopump was started, 20 min after arrest, the patient regained consciousness and became hemodynamically stable. He was transferred to the operating room and CABG was performed. The left-ventricular assistance by the Hemopump was started again to wean the patient from the cardiopulmonary bypass for better hemodynamics, and stopped after 30 min, i.e., 4 h after the initial cardiac arrest. One month later, the patient showed a small anteroseptal cicatricial myocardial infarction. Nevertheless, left ventricular function remained within normal limits.

Case 2: A 68-year-old man had severe double-vessel disease. His left-ventricular ejection fraction was 52%. Percutaneous transluminal angioplasty of the circumflex coronary artery was attempted. The procedure was complicated by circumflex coronary artery dissection, and cardiac arrest occurred. The patient was resuscitated during 1 h before the Hemopump was used. Under left-ventricular assistance by the Hemopump, spontaneous myocardial defibrillation was observed and the patient became hemodynamically stable, but he remained unconscious because of anesthesia or cerebral ischemia; the patient had no emergency CABG. The duration of the left-ventricular assistance was 4 days: the patient regained consciousness, there was no myocardial recuperation, and an antero-lateral myocardial infarction occurred. The patient could be weaned from the Hemopump on day 4, but he died on day 6 of infection and mesenteric infarction secondary to the initial cardiac low output.

Case 3: In this case, the indication was a cardiogenic shock 12 h after acute anteroseptal myocardial infarction in a 36-year-old woman. During the first 2 days, hemodynamic data were very good under left ventricular assistance by the Hemopump, but there was no sign of myocardial recuperation. The heart became more and more inefficient. On day 3, asystole occurred followed by a severe low cardiac output syndrome. The left-ventricular assistance by the Hemopump was not capable to support the circulation adequately at this time and we decided to implant a biventricular assistance (Abiomed) for 12 days before heart transplantation. This patient died 2 days after transplant from multi-organ failure.

Failure to wean from CPB

Case 4: A 46-year-old man underwent a left-ventricular aneurysm resection with a poor function of the remaining part of the left ventricle. The Hemopump was used to wean him from cardiopulmonary bypass. The duration of the left-ventricular assistance was 3 days and after myocardial recuperation, the patient could be weaned from the Hemopump with good hemodynamic result. Unfortunately, he died on day 4 of cerebral hemorrhage.

Cardiac allograft rejection

Case 5: A 47-year-old man developed a severe cardiac allograft rejection 2 years after a second heart transplantation performed 4 years after the first one. After cardiac arrest and successful resuscitation, the Hemopump was implanted. Hemodynamic variables were improved during support by the device. The allograft rejection was steroid and OKT3 resistant, and the patient died from multiorgan failure, before retransplantation, and after 8 days of circulatory support by the device.

Discussion

The duration of the Hemopump support ranged from 4 h to 8 days. The operative time required for device implantation, including confirming the position of the pump by fluoroscopy, was 25 min. All patients tolerated the implantation procedure, and none experienced surgical complications.

The hemodynamic status of each patient improved immediately after initiation of Hemopump support. There was no complication directly related to the use of the device and no drive shaft fractured.

Three of the five patients treated with the Hemopump could be weaned from the device. After removal of the device, all three patients remained hemodynamically stable. No clinical evidence of valvular damage or vascular injury was present, and no patients experienced thromboembolic episodes.

Four of the five patients treated by the Hemopump died. Two patients died after weaning from the Hemopump: one from a non-cardiac cause, and the second from organ failure secondary to the initial low output. The two other patients died because of low output during Hemopump support with a completely failing heart: one before heart retransplantation, and the second after replacement of an extracorporeal assist device followed by heart transplantation.

In fact, the Hemopump is a left-ventricular assist device, but cannot replace the left ventricle. The Hemopump seems to be a good technique of circulatory support for long duration left-ventricular assistance of a still working heart when possibility of myocardial recuperation exists: weaning from CPB, acute allograft failure. It is also a good technique for short-duration left-ventricular assistance of an inefficient heart as a bridge to emergency CABG after angioplasty failure, or as a bridge to angioplasty or CABG during acute myocardial infarction. But the Hemopump seems to be a poor technique for long-duration left-ventricular assistance of an inefficient heart when the hemodynamic output of the patient depends only on the Hemopump: In these cases, the capacity of the device in terms of high pump flows is too low, which renders the risk for irreversible multiorganfailure too high.

In conclusion, the Hemopump is a useful tool in the treatment of patients with potentially reversible cardiac failure.

References

1. Duncan JM, Frazier OH, Radovancevic B, et al. (1989) Implantation techniques for the Hemopump. Ann Thorac Surg 48: 733–735
2. Frazier OH, Wampler RK, Ducan JM, et al. (1990) First human use of the Hemopump, a catheter-mounted ventricular assist device. Ann Thorac Surg 49: 299–304
3. Loisance D, Dubois-Rande JL, Deleuze Ph et al. (1990) Prophylactic intraventricular pumping in high-risk coronary angioplasty. Lancet 335: 438–440
4. Wampler RK, Moise JC, Frazier OH et al. (1988) In vivo evaluation of a peripheral vascular access axial flow blood pump. ASAIO Transac 34: 450–454

Hemopump for supported angioplasty

D. Loisance, J.L. Dubois-Rande, Ph. Deleuze, O. Rosenval, J. Okude, F. Wan, N. Shiiya, H. Geschwind

Centre Hospitalier Henri Mondor, Faculté de Médicine, Creteil, France

Introduction

A new approach in the management of extremely sick patients with unstable myocardial ischaemia selected for coronary angioplasty has been recently proposed (2). It is based on mechanical assistance of the left ventricle, obtained by intra-ventricular implantation of the Hemopump. The prophylactic implantation of this new type of intra-ventricular pump, prior to the coronary angioplasty itself, should reduce the risk and the consequences of sudden cardiac arrest during the procedure. The present report of the first nine cases performed at Henri-Mondor's Hospital clearly shows the benefit and limitations of the technique.

Protocol

1) The whole approach is based on the use of the Hemopump. This new (3) arterial pump is based on the principle of the Archimedes screw and consists of an inlet cannula, an axial-flow blood pump, a drive cable contained in a polymer sheath, and a rotor. The pump head is in a 21F cannula; it is activated by a rotating electromagnetic field. The spiral veins of the pump head, which rotates at a very high speed – 20000 to 25000 rpm/min – permit the displacement of blood from the tip of the cannula, placed in the left ventricular cavity, to the outflow port of the cannula in the ascending aorta. Flow rates may be adjusted from 0 up to 3.–3.5 l/min. Insertion into the ventricle of the cannula is made under fluoroscopic control, via the femoral artery.

2) The technique of implantation has been considerably simplified in comparison to the technique originally proposed (3). A silicone occluder was designed at the Centre de Recherches Chirurgicales to permit occlusion of the aortic orifice of the cannula, through which blood may regurgitate during the femoral insertion (Fig. 1). This occluder allows the insertion via the femoral artery, without implantation of a dacron graft. Under local anesthesia, the common femoral artery is exposed and inspected. A guide wire is first inserted into the left ventricle under fluoroscopic control. It will facilitate the rapid positioning of the cannula into the ventricle. The femoral artery is occluded, 5 cm upstream of the level of the arteriotomy, around the entry of the guide wire. The cannula is then inserted into the femoral artery, until its whole orifice is in the vessel. The femoral artery is then unclamped and the cannula pushed into the aorta. The occluder is removed as the drive cable is inserted. A few separate prolene sutures permit to close the arteriotomy around the drive cable.

The tip of the cannula is positioned in the ventricle. The pump is activated, delete as soon as the tip of the cannula is in the ascending aorta.

3) Immediately prior to cannula insertion, a Swan-Ganz catheter is placed into the pulmonary artery. Cardiac output is measured by the thermodilution technique. Routine

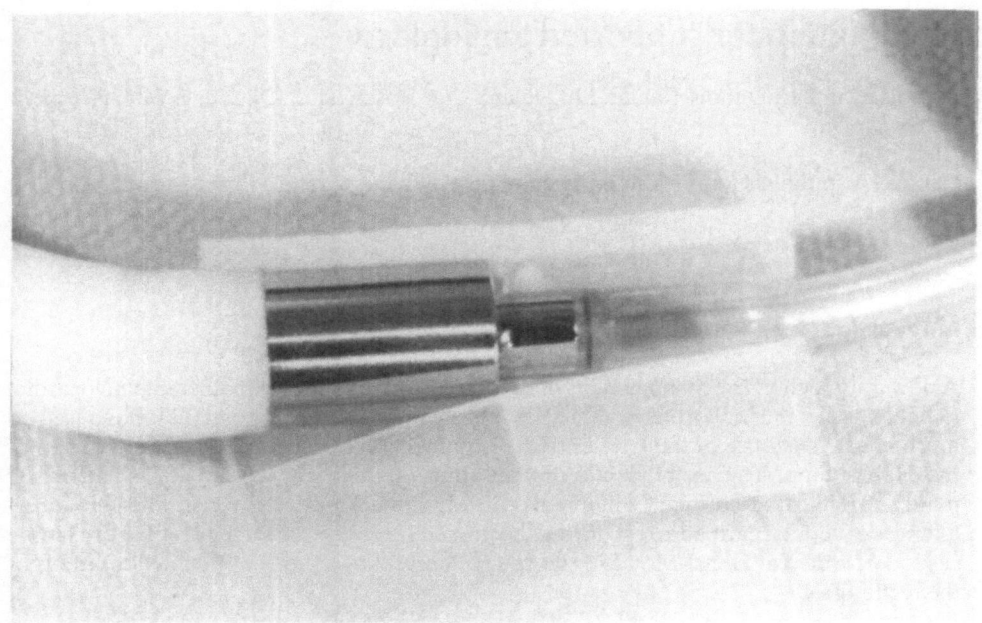

Fig. 1. The silicone occluder, used during the implantation.

hemodynamic indices and parameters are continuously monitored and computed. As the pump is activated, at maximal speed, PTCA is performed, using the conventional technique. Inflation time is 3 min, at a 6–10 ATA pressure, three times for each stenosis.

Premedication includes aspirin (250 mg per day, starting 2 days pre-operatively), and heparin (1 mg/kg at time of implantation of the Hemopump) is maintained for 24 h, the clotting time being kept twice the control level.

Clinical experience

Criteria for inclusion into the protocol are as follows: evolving acute myocardial ischemia, unresponsive to any medical therapy, related to a significant stenosis with a patent distal run off in a patient which cannot be operated without a major operative risk or dilated wihout any risk, because of clinical or anatomical characteristics. Nine patients were selected for the procedure from February 1989 to February 1990. The contra-indications for surgery were: previous surgery in five patients (twice in two), with no venous or arterial material suitable for grafting, low ejection fraction and poor ventricle in six. Table 1, which summarizes the anatomical coronary condition of these patients clearly shows that in every case the culprit lesions were localized on the only patent vessel. Age itself has never been considered as a contra-indication for surgery.

The pump has been successfully implanted in six patients. A typical case is shown in Fig. 2. In two patients (numbers 3 and 7), the size of the iliac artery did not allow insertion of the cannula and in one (number 8), the tortuous iliac artery did not allow progression of the cannula. For patient number 3 the PTCA was nevertheless, performed. The vessel

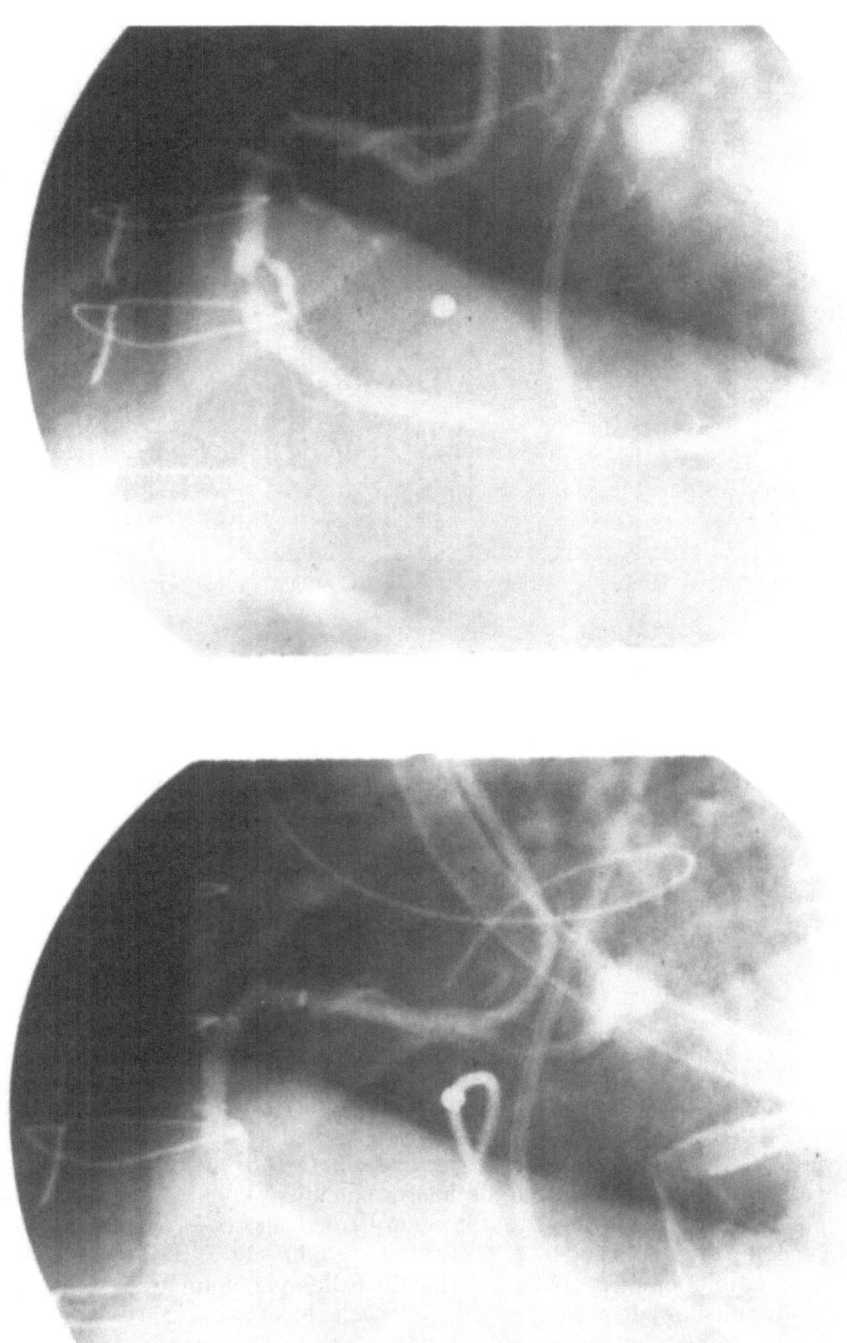

Fig. 2. Coronary angiography prior to (1a) and following (1b) supported PTCA. The left main coronary artery is totally occluded and perfusion of both ventricles is given by the right artery only.

Table 1. Coronary status prior to PTCA (LAD = Left anterior descending artery, Cir = circumflex artery, Sten = Stenosis, occl = occlusion).

Case	Left main	LAD lesion	LAD status run off	CIR lesion	CIR status run off	RC lesion	RC status run off	CABG nb	CABG on	CABG status	Culprit lesion
1	–	100%	+	95%	±	100%	–	2	LAD RC	open occl	circ
2	occl	100%	0	100%	0	95%	±	–	–	–	RC
3	–	95%	+	100%	0	100%	–	–	–	–	LAD
4	occl	100%	0	100%	0	95%	+	3	marg LAD Right	occl occl occl	RC
5	–	100%	0	95%	+	100%	0	1	LAD	occl	circ
6	–	100%	0	95%	+	100%	0	–	–	–	circ
7	95%	50%	+	0%	+	100%	0	–	–	–	L.main
8	95%	95%	+	0%	±	100%	0	1	LAD marg	open occl	marg
9	–	100%	–	95%	+	100%	–		LAD RC marg	occl occl occl	circ

Legend: LAD = left anterior descending – circ = circumflex – RC = right coronary – marg = marginal – L. main = left main

Status of run off: + = good – 0 = absent – ± = infiltrated lesions expressed in %

Table 2. Hemodynamics pre and post PTCA, and during off/on maneuvers of the Hemopump (PCWP = pulmonary capillary wedged in mmHg pressure, CI = cardiac index).

Case	PCWP Pre	PCWP Post	Pump flow L/min	CI-L/min/m² Pre	CI-L/min/m² Post
1	18	14	3.4	1.6	2.4
2	16	13	3.6	2.0	2.6
4	7	7	3.1	2.2	2.7
5	12	8	3.2	2.4	2.5
6	19	15	3.1	2.6	2.8

was successfully re-opened; a re-occlusion occured 5 min later, and the patient died despite new attempts at reperfusion. In the six other patients, dilatation was performed successfully.

During the PTCA, hemodynamic changes have been observed (Table 2) showing a definite improvement in the left-ventricular mechanical condition. Pump flow ranged from 2.4 to 3.5 l/min. Cardiac index increased as the pump was activated by an average of 23%. Capillary wedged pressure dropped by 17%. The most striking observation was the lack of any clinical deterioration of the patient during the balloon inflation itself. Nevertheless, ECG monitoring showed a prolonged atrio ventricular block in one and a ventricular tachycardia in four, with a spontaneous return to normal sinus rythm after a few minutes.

Late follow-up showed successful results in the six patients. Five patients, are under medical therapy, symptom-free, 12–24 months following the episode of acute ischemia and PTCA. One patient has been selected for an elective surgical revascularization after disappearance of the myocardial ischaemia. He is now asymptomatic.

Discussion

1) The present clinical experience clearly supports the concept of prophylactic, non-invasive mechanical ventricular assistance for patients selected for high-risk PTCA. Simplicity, safety, and efficacy of the method based on the Hemopump are now well documented. The use of a specially designed occluder permits to avoid massive bleeding during the time of implantation as does the use of a side graft proposed by Frazier. This experience differs drastically from other approaches based on more invasive methods of ventricular support such as the systems using extra corporeal veno-arterial shunting. These systems require a full heparinization of the patient, sophisticated equipments and trained pump technicians. They also induce, as in every extra corporeal circulation, deleterious effects such as complement activation, thrombocytopenia, and coagulation diasthesis. Finally, these systems do not allow a complete left-ventricular unloading.

The already obvious benefits of the Hemopump should be even more spectacular when new designs of pump, based on the same principle become available. The most appealing improvement will be the possibility of a percutaneous implantation of the cannula. Nevertheless, the most dramatic one will be the higher flow rate of the pump, permitting a complete left-ventricular support.

2) The mechanism of the reduction of the risk of the PTCA itself is probably complex. The most significant change induced by the Hemopump procedure is probably the drop in the left-ventricular dimensions and external work. This leads to a drop in the myocardial energy requirements which is clinically helpful during balloon inflation. A second mechanism may be found in the improvement of the perfusion, through the non-occluded vessels and the collateral vessels. Analysis of the changes in the myocardial perfusion and function deserves more specific study, and is presently under way (1).

3) Introduction of the Hemopump technique in intensive care units will change the strategies in the most critically ill patients. It should permit a very early decompression of the left ventricle in massive myocardial infarction. Consequently, the chances of a real recovery of the ischemic non-infarcted areas will be enhanced. A reduction in the need of urgent cardiac replacement or invasive methods of support to the failing heart should be investigated.

References

1. Dubois Randé JL, Zelinsky R, Deleuze Ph, Geschwind H, Loisance D (1991) Coronary hemo-dynamics during Hemopump left ventricular assistance. Int J Artif organs (in press)
2. Loisance D, Dubois Randé JL, Deleuze Ph, Okudé J, Rosenval O, Geschwind H (1990) Prophylactic intraventricular pumping in high risk coronary angiography. Lancet 335: 438–440
3. Wampler RK, Moise JC, Frazier OH, Olsen DB (1988) In vivo evaluation of a peripheral vascular – Access axial flow blood pump. ASAIO Transactions 34: 450–454

Indications for the use of the Hemopump

W. Flameng

University Clinic Gasthuisberg, Department of Cardiac Surgery, Leuven, Belgium

Introduction

The indication for the use of a left-ventricular assist system is, in principle, that of an untreatable low cardiac output state related to a severe degree of cardiac failure. Cardiac failure however is a very complex feature which is based on a large variety of pathophysiological mechanisms. Complete global akinesia of the left ventricle after extended cardiac surgery, for example, may be due to post ischemic myocardial stunning and will be entirely reversible provided the circulation remains temporarily supported.

On the other hand, cardiogenic shock may be related to an end-stage chronic cardiomyopathy, refractory to any medical treatment. Long-term mechanical support of these hearts will not result in recovery of cardiac function. Therefore, in patients suffering from cardiac failure, the decision to apply mechanical support and the choice of the type of support device itself will be directly related to the pathophysiological background of the actual low cardiac output state. Furthermore, not only the underlying disease of the myocardium, but also certain technical limitations of a given support system will define the indication for the use of a specific device.

Finally, some limitations must be considered which are not related in the first place to the system or device, but to the associated disease of the patient himself. In patients with peripheral vascular disease for example the Hemopump may be difficult to introduce.

General principles

A *first principle* for successful use of the Hemopump is that of *partial assistance*. When the impairment of the left ventricle is complete, a more powerful system is required which is able to totally replace cardiac function. Left-ventricular function, although severely depressed may not be completely absent because the maximum flow capacities of this type of axial pump is only 3.5 liter per minute, at optimal conditions of peripheral resistance (8). The Hemopump is a device with *moderate support* capacities.

The basic mechanism of such partial loss of left-ventricular function may be manifold. Acute ischemia is the most frequent cause of myocardial failure, and without timely reperfusion complete loss of function will be definite. Upon reperfusion, however, a temporary phase of ventricular dysfunction will remain. This phenomenon is referred to as myocardial stunning (1). The underlying mechanism of this type of postischemic dysfunction is still unclear. It seems not to be a problem of myocardial energy production (2), but rather of energy utilization. Nevertheless, stunning is a temporary phenomenon which is completely reversible provided perfusion persists. This is an indication for temporary support of the circulation. Indeed, typical for myocardial stunning is its reversibility. Recovery of function is delayed and the delay can be extended to 1 week or more (6). This leads to the *second principle* of Hemopump assist: that of *reversibility* of myocardial dysfunction. The fundamental condition for the use of an axial assist system in the form as it exists at present is that the depression of left-ventricular function must be expected to be reversible after sustained reperfusion. In general practice, prediction of reversibility of postischemic dysfunction is difficult. Indeed, there is still no reliable correlate of function recovery after ischemic insult. Usually, global ischemia in the presence of normal coronary arteries, induced by cross clamping of the aorta in routine cardiac surgery is not severe enough to produce extended necrosis and irreversible cardiac failure when some degree of hypothermia was associated. In most cases ischemia-induced myocardial necrosis occurs in the presence of coronary artery disease when revascularization and reperfusion of the coronary system is either incomplete or extremely retarded. In cases of evolving myocardial infarction a critical ischemic interval of 4–6 h was suggested (4). However, time of the ischemic interval is not the only determinant of the extent of myocardial necrosis in the presence of a coronary artery occlusion (3, 5). Also, the extent of the perfusion area of the blocked coronary artery and the degree of development of coronary collateral vessels will define the final amount of myocardial necrosis (5). In case of cardiogenic shock due to an evolving myocardial infarction in a non-surgical patient, the use of a Hemopump is not only indicated because of its ability to support the circulation, but also because of its unloading properties. Unloading of the left ventricle reduces oxygen consumption of the myocardium which is also a factor influencing the final size of the infarction (5).

A *third principle* for the successful use of a left-ventricular assist device is its ability to deliver *adequate regional organ blood flow* distribution. In the experimental study of Wouters et al. (see Chapter 4), it is shown that the Hemopump system is capable of providing adequate organ perfusion to all vital organs. However, as also shown in a previous study of Sukehiro et al. (7) when using a centrifugal pump as an assist device, blood flow to the kidney is very susceptible to conditions of cardiogenic shock. Although renal blood flow can be restored during mechanical support, some decrease in renal flow was observed after weaning from the device. In clinical practice, *long-lasting multi-organ failure* has a severe negative impact on outcome after circulatory support.

A *fourth principle* for the use of the Hemopump is its limitation of use only in *isolated left-ventricular failure*. It is obvious from the actual construction of the Hemopump that only the left circulation can be supported by this system. Therefore, the indication of the Hemopump remains limited to cases of failure of the left heart. Although it may be difficult to differentiate between isolated left failure and biventricular heart failure, careful analysis of hemodynamic data combined with transoesophagal echocardiography will allow diagnosis of participation of the right ventricle.

Specific indications for the use of the Hemopump

In *non-surgical* patients the Hemopump can be used for *prevention of low cardiac ouput* during PTCA procedures in high-risk patients. The device was successfully used in patients undergoing complex PTCA procedures (see Chapter 9).

In medically treated patients suffering from an evolving *myocardial infarction* associated with cardiogenic shock the circulation can be supported by the Hemopump. As mentioned above, the general principles of correct indication should be respected. At first, the left ventricle should not be completely deteriorated. The device should not be used in any reanimation procedure. Second, some degree of reversibility should be expected. This means that reperfusion of the blocked coronary artery should be induced by thrombolysis and that reperfusion should be obtained timely i.e., within 4 h after onset of symptoms. Furthermore, the diagnosis of isolated left heart failure must be clear. Occlusion of a dominant right coronary artery may result in extended infarction of the right ventricle. At present clinical experience with the Hemopump in patients suffering from low cardiac output due to myocardial infarction is scarce. A randomized clinical trial comparing the effects of the Hemopump with those of intra-aortic balloon counterpulsation is needed.

The most extensive experience with the use of the Hemopump is available in *postcardiotomy low cardiac output state*. Figure 1 shows a schematic presentation of the indication for the use of the Hemopump in postcardiotomy patients suffering from low cardiac output.

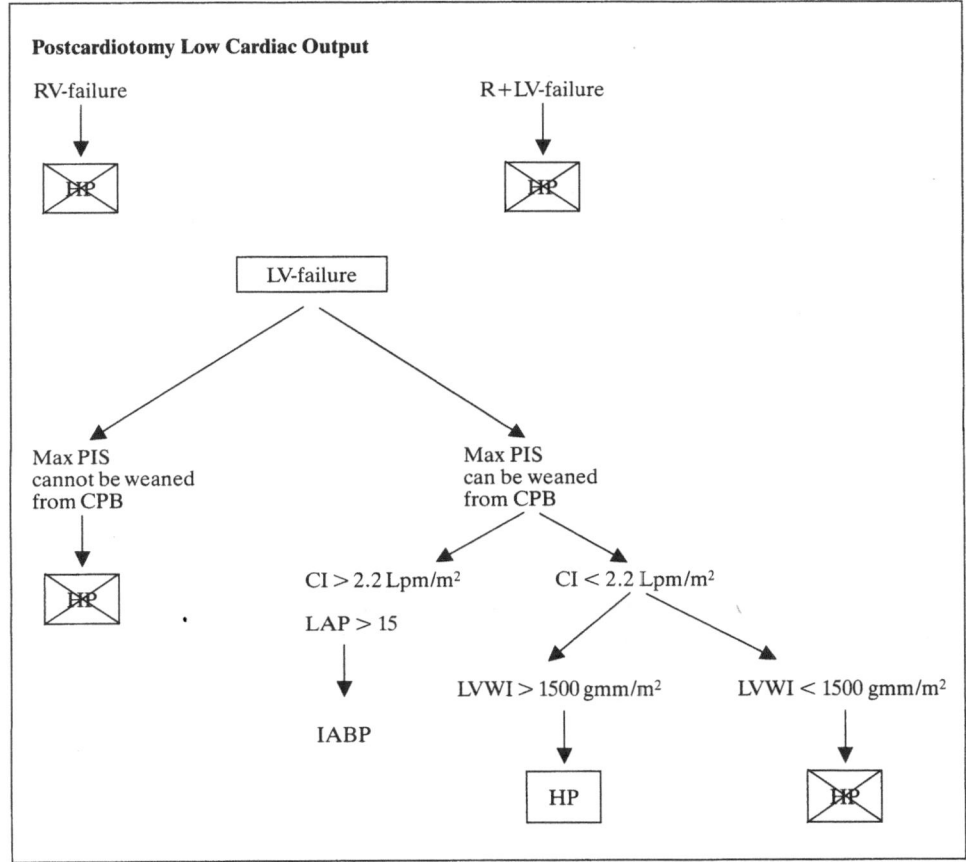

Fig. 1: Indication for the use of the hemopump in postcardiotomy low cardiac output. RV: Right ventricle; LV: left ventricle; PIS: positive inotropic support; CPB: cardiopulmonary bypass; HP: Hemopump; CI: cardiac index; LVWI: left-ventricular work index.

At first, the diagnosis of isolated left heart failure is made. When isolated right-heart failure, or a combination of right and left heart failure are present, the Hemopump is not used, and a paracorporeal assist system may be indicated.

In case of isolated left-heart failure, the Hemopump is also not to be used when the patient cannot be weaned from cardiopulmonary bypass, in spite of maximal positive inotropic support. In this case again a paracorporeal assist system may be indicated. When, however, the patient can be weaned from cardiopulmonary bypass during maximal positive inotropic support, but rapidly develops a low cardiac output state, the decision to use a Hemopump depends upon the hemodynamic parameters, mainly cardiac index and left-ventricular stroke work index. When cardiac index is below 2.2 Lpm/m^2 and LVSW I is below 1500 gmm/m^2, no Hemopump is used, and the only solution again may be a paracorporeal support device. When LVSWI, however, is larger than 1500 gmm/m^2, the Hemopump may be the device of first choice. When CI is above 2.2 Lpm/m^2, but the left atrial pressure increases to pathological values (>15 mm Hg) an intraaortic ballon counter-pulsation can be useful in a first attempt. When no improvement is obtained, the IABP can be replaced by the more efficient Hemopump.

There is only a limited experience with the use of the Hemopump as a *bridge to transplantation*. In our series where the Hemopump was used as a bridge to transplantation three out of four patients could be transplanted succesfully.

Nevertheless, the first option for the use of the Hemopump should be to use it in theoretically reversible forms of cardiac failure. The main reason is that this kind of axial pump system is of limited power and cannot totally replace the left heart. In case of bridging, it might be that left-ventricular function deteriorates completely and irreversibly, a situation which cannot be dealt with by the Hemopump. A second aspect is that the time span for bridging can extend considerably when a suitable donor heart is not available. At the moment, the time limits for the use of an Hemopump are still unknown and extended periods of assist may be complicated by hemolytic and mechanical difficulties. Currently, the Hemopump has become a bridge-to-transplantation device when, unexpectedly the heart does not recover as it was originally expected to do so.

Limitations and prognostic considerations

There are a number of limitations to the present Hemopump system which are related to the device itself.

First, there is the limited flow capacity of the system (3.5 liter/min) which makes it unsuitable for patients with a large body surface area , who require a large fraction of cardiac output to be supplied by the device. Only in case of moderate reduction of cardiac function, will the maximum rate of assisted flow be sufficient to produce an overall output, capable of maintaining adequate organ flow distribution in these patients.

The size of the cannula (21F) may be too large to allow introduction of the device via the femoral artery in small-sized patients. An alternative in this respect is the approach via the iliac artery, but this does not simplify the procedure. Also, the presence of atherosclerotic lesions and plaques in the peripheral vasculature may make the insertion of the cannula impossible. The presence of an artificial valve in aortic position will be a contra-indication for the use of the Hemopump, because the cannula cannot be entered into the left ventricle without disturbing valve function.

The presence of an adhesive thrombus in the left ventricle is also a clear contra-indication because of the danger of inducing emboli after insertion of the tube into the ventricular cavity.

Patients with known abnormalities of their blood elements are not suited for the use of the Hemopump, because the system has the potential to destroy platelets and red blood cells.

Conclusion

In summary, the Hemopump is a non-invasive and efficient left-ventricular assist system of moderate power. Indications are limited to isolated left-ventricular failure, which is incomplete and reversible.

References

1. Braunveld E, Kloner RA (1982) The stunned myocardium: Prolonged, postischemic ventricular dysfunction. Circulation 66: 1146–1149
2. Flameng W, Andres J, Ferdinande P, Mattheussen M, Van Belle H (1991) Mitochondrial fuction in myocardial stunning. J, Mol, Cell, Cardiol, 23: 1–11
3. Flameng W, Lesaffre E, Vanhaecke J (1990) Determinants of infarct size in non-human primates. Basic res cardiol 85: 392–403
4. Flameng W, Sergeant P, Vanhaecke J, Suy R (1987) Emergency coronary bypass grafting for evolving myocardial infarction: effects on infarct size and left ventricular function. J Thorac Cardiovasc Surg 94/1: 124–31
5. Flameng W, Vanhaecke J, Lesaffre E (1989) Limitations of experimental infarct size by drugs. J cardiovasc pharmacol 14 (Suppl 9): S29–S33
6. Heyndrickx GR, Baig H, Nelkins P, Leusen K, Fishbein MC, Vatner SF (1978) Depression of regional blood flow and wall thickening after brief coronary occlusions. An J Physiol 234: H653–H659
7. Sukehiro S, Flameng W (1990) Effects of left ventricular assist for cardiogenic shock on cardiac function and organ blood flow distribution. Ann thorac surg 50: 374–383
8. Wampler RK (1987) Investigator's manual for clinical investigations of the Nimbres Hemopump. Nimbres Medical, Inc. Rancho Cordova, California. Doc. nr. 2005301

M. **Kaltenbach**, R. E. **Vliestra**

Concise Cardiology

1991. 180 pp. with 120 figures, 10 tables.
Hardcover DM 60,–. ISBN 3-7985-0864-X

This volume covers the wide range of disciplines in cardiology, and it includes thorough clinical disease-recognition profiles, as well as concise descriptions of therapy methods. Special diagnostic considerations and problems in the management of cardiac and circulatory diseases are discussed, and the information is presented in a logical order. The text has practical significance for both review and for teaching, and the work emphasizes understanding of the material as opposed to just memorization.

Wide acceptance of this work has been demonstrated by the success of the first two German-language editions, authored by Martin Kaltenbach; this first English-language edition represents a cooperation with the American cardiologist R. E. Vlietstra.

K. R. **Karsch**, K. K. **Haase** (Eds.)

Coronary Laser Angioplasty. An Update

1991. X, 182 pp with 98 figures. Hardcover DM 89,–.
ISBN 3-7985-0882-8

Coronary Excimer Laser Angioplasty was introduced about two years ago for the clinical treatment of patients with coronary heart disease. Its present status and a critical analysis based on experiences with this method are the focal points of this volume.

This is the first compendium written on this still relatively new interventional method and it details the basic techniques of Laser Excimer Angioplasty. In addition to providing an overview of laser-tissue interactions, it also describes the currently available application systems.

The authors of this work are from leading international centers where this intracoronary treatment method was developed.

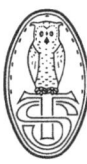

Steinkopff Dr. Dietrich Steinkopff Verlag
Saalbaustraße 12, 6100 Darmstadt/FRG

N. **Friedel**, R. **Hetzer**, D. **Royston** (Eds.)

Blood Use in Cardiac Surgery

1991. X. 282 pp. Cloth DM 98.–. ISBN 3-7985-0841-0.

> The development of cardiac surgery to its present state would not have been possible without blood substitution by homologous donor blood. This volume presents a consensus from clinicians and researchers for improving and developing present blood-saving measures in order to minimize blood loss and transfusion risks.

H. O. **Vetter**, R. **Hetzer**, H. **Schmutzler** (Eds.)

Ischemic Mitral Incompetence

1991. XII. 212 pp., Cloth DM 74.–. ISBN 0-7985-0799-6.

> Ischemic Mitral Incompetence provides a review of the current knowledge of mitral valve insufficiency. Diagnostic techniques and indications for surgical interventions, particularly, coronary bypass operation, valve reconstruction, and mitral replacement are presented by leading international practitioners.

U. J. **Winter**, N. **Treese**, K. **Wassermann**, H. W. **Höpp** (Eds.)

Computerized Cardiopulmonary Exercise Testing (CPX)

1991. 202 pp. Cloth DM 84,–. ISBN 3-7985-0859-3.

> This volume presents contributions by international experts on the current diagnostic possibilities of modern, noninvasive, computerized cardiopulmonary exercise testing (CPX) in cardiopulmonary disease.

H. **Drexler**, A. M. **Zeiher**, E. **Bassenge**, H. **Just** (Eds.)

Endothelial Mechanisms of Vasomotor Control

With Special Reference to the Coronary Circulation
1991. 352 pp. Hardcover DM 98,–. ISBN 3-7985-0866-6.

> In order to maintain the fluidity of the blood and the patency of the blood vessels, the endothelial cells support remarkable functions. Their structure, function under normal conditions, and dysfunction of the dilator mechanism are the main topics of this book.

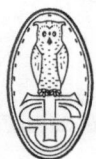

Steinkopff Dr. Dietrich Steinkopff Verlag
Saalbaustraße 12, 6100 Darmstadt/FRG